Communicating in Sign

Creative Ways to Learn
American Sign Language (ASL)

Written by Diane P. Chambers
with Lee Ann Chearney

Edited by D. Keith Robertson
Illustrations by Paul M. Setzer

With an Introduction by Bernard Bragg

A Flying Hands Book

Produced by Amaranth

A Fireside Book
Published by Simon & Schuster

FIRESIDE
Rockefeller Center
1230 Avenue of the Americas
New York, NY 10020

Produced by Amaranth
379 8th Street
Brooklyn, New York 11215

Design by Publisher's Studio
4 Airline Drive
Albany, New York 12205

Deaf community diagram appearing on page 53, reprinted by permission of the publisher, in
C. Baker-Shenk, D. Cokely, *American Sign Language: A Teacher's Resource Text on Grammar and
Culture,* (Washington, D.C.: Gallaudet University Press, 1991), 56. Copyright 1991 by Gallaudet
University.

Photographs in this book appear by courtesy of the Gallaudet University Photography
Department. Special thanks to the Office of Public Relations, and to Mike Kaika, Director of
Media Relations, at Gallaudet University for assistance in captioning the photos.

Manufactured in the United States of America

10   9   8   7   6   5   4   3   2

Library of Congress Cataloging-in-Publication Data

Chambers, Diane P.
    Communicating in sign : creative ways to learn American Sign Language (ASL) / written
  by Diane P. Chambers, with Lee Ann Chearney; edited by D. Keith Robertson; illustrations by
  Paul M. Setzer; with an introduction by Bernard Bragg.
      p.   cm. — (A flying hands book)
    Includes bibliographical references and index.
    1. American Sign Language.   I. Chearney, Lee Ann   II. Amaranth (Brooklyn, N.Y.)
  III. Title. IV. Series.
  HV2474.C43   1998
  419—dc21   97-51145
  ISBN 0-684-83520-7   CIP

Acknowledgments

My heartfelt gratitude and respect to D. Keith Robertson and Ruthie Rowan for teaching my hands to fly; to YaYa for inspiring me; and to Linda, David, Paul, and my extended family and faithful friends for their encouragement and support.

Many thanks to Lee Ann Chearney at Amaranth for her patience and belief in this project, to Sarah Baker at Fireside, and to Candace Levy for her remarkable copyediting skills.

Flying Hands shows special gratitude to Paul M. Setzer and Mike Kaika whose talents and work have been invaluable.

Grateful acknowledgment to the Deaf models who posed for Paul Setzer's wonderful illustrations.

My thanks and admiration to the Deaf community whose language and culture are celebrated in this book.

—Diane P. Chambers

FOR MY PARENTS,
whose spirits live on

Contents

Note to the Reader

American Sign Language (ASL) is a beautifully visual and expressive language—a different language from the English language. Gender pronouns, "she" and "he," are most readily understood through the *visual*. For this reason, gender pronouns are used differently in ASL than they are in English. In spoken and written English, however, gender pronouns cannot be communicated easily as visual concepts, leading to unfortunate, and often unintended, gender-biased usage.

To avoid ascribing any gender significance to ASL signs, the decision was made to use a gender-neutral pronoun in the English text of *Communicating in Sign*. So, instead of reading "she" and "he," readers will find "their" used as both the singular and plural pronoun. This usage is gaining acceptability in English as an alternative for writers and speakers who do not want to arbitrarily assign gender to a pronoun in a sentence. By assigning a gender-neutral pronoun, we preserve the visual focus of conversing in ASL and put the correct, predominant emphasis on the noun instead of the gender pronoun.

Introduction

In the 1960's, I developed a theory called Visual Vernacular—a form of mime using cinematic techniques that is very much part of American Sign Language (ASL). As I was involved with the National Theater of the Deaf, and also many years afterward as an independent performer, I was able to expose many people all over the world to this theatrical mode of expression.

Since the days of civil rights liberation in America, the Deaf community has been striving to show itself to the general public as a people having their own language, culture, and self-esteem. *Communicating in Sign: Creative Ways to Learn American Sign Language (ASL)*, I am pleased to say, furthers this effort. Fittingly named, Flying Hands has developed a way to lead people through the exciting role of learning a new language: ASL!

Like any other language in the world, ASL has evolved since the early days of our Founding Fathers. A mystery to many, it is lately becoming less so thanks to an ever-growing number of books on Deaf people and their language and culture. The Flying Hands method is unique in that it includes not only the vocabulary and sophisticated points of ASL grammar and syntax but also a comprehensive introduction to the Deaf world. For example, such questions are clearly answered: How do Deaf people communicate on the phone and use alarm clocks? Or what is proper etiquette? Without a doubt, people involved in any profession and setting will find this book invaluable.

Flying Hands's creative approach makes it the definitive guide to learning the language and culture of Deaf people. I highly recommend it to any person who is interested in associating and working with Deaf people.

Five years ago, I attended the homecoming event at Gallaudet University. Many Deaf students and alumni from all over the world gathered for the occasion. Keith Robertson, a Deaf alumnus, recognized me and began a conversation with me in ASL. He expressed his concern about how best to help people who are interested in learning ASL. As he had been teaching ASL for several years, he was well aware of the challenges many hearing people face in learning sign language.

The Deaf community is a tightly knit group of resolute people who have struggled together to empower themselves. We have made many efforts and successes in bridging the communication gap between the Deaf and Hearing cultures. *Communicating in Sign* is one of those successes. Diane P. Chambers, president of Flying Hands, has met the challenging task of writing a book that introduces a wide variety of professionals and laypeople to ASL and Deaf culture. Keith's input as a member of the Deaf community fulfills his desire to help Hearing people appreciate the Deaf world. People working in such fields as hotel and restaurant management, retail stores, communications, service organizations, education, finance, management, theater arts, etc., will be absolutely intrigued by this book.

Finally, here is a book that leads us into a new experience through American Sign Language.

My congratulations to you, Diane. Your dream has taken shape and your book will fly!

—Bernard Bragg, 1998

Emotions

American Sign Language (ASL) is a beautiful language full of emotions. When we speak, we use our vocal chords, tongue, mouth, and ears. When we sign we use our hands, eyes, lips, jaw, and sense of touch. Our sense of touch, our feeling sense, springs to life when we sign. As we make the signs for emotions, we are really expressing how these emotions touch our body and our soul. If we are hungry, if we are happy, these basic feeling states easily transcend the spoken word. Learning to express emotions in American Sign Language is the key to understanding its power and immediacy.

The Five Basic Components of ASL

Imagine that you cannot speak or hear. You must find a way to communicate your feelings to others. Immediately, the almost unconscious physical responses to emotions that our bodies naturally make become our most basic vehicle for expression, instead of merely enhancing the words we speak. These physical responses are sometimes so second

1

nature to us that we do not even realize our bodies communicate as strongly as our words. The band Extreme has a song that asks what someone would do to show she or he cared if the words *I love you* were taken away. To show love in ASL, we must speak it without words—at least without words as we know them. The five components of American Sign Language come from the ways we can use our bodies to communicate and from our powers of observation to understand whatever emotion is communicated to us. The five components, in order of importance, are:

1. Eye contact
2. Facial expression
3. Body language
4. Mouth movements
5. Hand movements

Eye Contact. Communication is impossible unless your partner is looking at you. Looking away signals the end to a conversation and can be a great source of distress for the speaker if she or he is interrupted or distracted unexpectedly by a break in eye contact. Breaking eye contact is often a sign of anger or rudeness.

Maintaining eye contact is so important to communicating successfully in ASL that, within the Deaf culture, it is inappropriate to sign "Excuse me" when inadvertently disturbing a conversation between two other people. To draw their attention away by focusing it on your own interloping presence is considered more intrusive than simply moving along as quickly and unobtrusively as possible.

Hearing people must make a special effort to understand the importance of eye contact and a Deaf person's reliance on it. For example, a hearing student can listen to the teacher while taking notes or even while looking out the window. A Deaf student must watch a sign language interpreter to understand what the teacher is saying (or watch while the teacher signs).

Facial Expression. Facial expressions convey adjectives, adverbs, intensity, superlatives, and even denote pronouns through head movements toward or away from someone. Think about it. Is the person driving the car spaced out, sleepy, or fully attentive? Facial expressions comment on the action conveyed or present the opinion of the speaker in relation to it. For example, if you are unhappy that your little brother has a larger portion of chocolate ice cream than you do, your expression would show dismay as you nod toward him and sign the sentence, "He has more chocolate ice cream."

Body Language. Our bodies react naturally to the stimuli presented by the world around us. We move away from things we don't like or that we fear. We approach things we are curious about or are attracted to. Simple observation of another person's instinctive movement toward or away from outside stimuli can speak volumes about his or her true feelings. In ASL, these body movements are incorporated into the performance of signs to give richness and depth to the concepts communicated.

Mouth Movements. Mouth movements in sign language don't necessarily mean English words formed by the lips. Grammatically, mouth movements can depict sizes and shapes. For example, when referring to a wide or large object, the speaker blows out his or her cheeks. When referring to a thin or small object, like a piece of wire, the speaker purses the lips or sucks air in.

Hand Movements. The formal signs or hand movements of ASL cannot be separated from the four preceding components of the language. All components are essential for fluent conversation. ASL is a language based on relationships in space and pictorial concepts, not on English words. It is important to remember that formal ASL signs are not always strict synonyms for English words, strung together to form sentences in exactly the same manner. As English is the first language for most of us, the transition to ASL can be difficult and will require some special effort. As in many other foreign languages, one sign in ASL can mean several different things, depending on facial expression, body language, or any of the other essential components.

As you learn to communicate in sign, it is important to embrace its physicality, its visual beauty and movement. Hearing people are often taught from childhood that it is not polite to express emotion graphically in public settings. The well-chosen word substitutes for the body that quakes inwardly with unspoken emotion. A blank-faced expression does nothing to promote communication with Deaf people. As we learn to become less inhibited about showing the way we feel and as we worry less and less about so-called proper or improper ways to express ourselves, the richness of communicating emotions in ASL will add depth to our very understanding of what it means to feel each precious human emotion. Exploring the ways that emotions touch us will help us empathize with others and make strong emotional connections to them.

Feeling Emotions with Your Body

Using your hands, face, and body to communicate is called *nonverbal communication*. In this way, you begin to think in pictures and three dimensions instead of English words.

Let's begin. Below you will find a list of ten emotional states. Think about how you feel whenever you experience each emotion.

- Fear
- Anger
- Surprise
- Shock
- Happiness

- Sadness
- Tiredness
- Frustration
- Amusement
- Excitement

Now, read the list again. Stop at each word and concentrate on the natural movements your body, face, and hands make when you feel this emotion. With a partner, or in front of a mirror, try to demonstrate each one. Let's compare your interpretations to the way most people naturally react to the emotions listed and to the way dictionaries define the experience of each. Common facial expressions are illustrated.

Fear n. *A distressing emotion caused by an anticipation or awareness of danger; a feeling of dread or apprehension.* v. *To be afraid.*

Our natural reaction is to lean away from something that makes us afraid. Sometimes we get a butterfly feeling in our stomachs and a tightening in our lungs. When we experience fear and show it, our bodies tend to lean away, shoulders back, eyes looking directly at or above the frightening thing, jaws tightening, and the head tilting back. Practice this several times in front of a mirror. Remember, however, the most important aspect here is to experience the emotion and feel the body's natural reaction. Imagine that Martians have invaded Earth, as did millions of frightened Americans during the 1938 Orson Welles radio broadcast of *The War of the Worlds.*

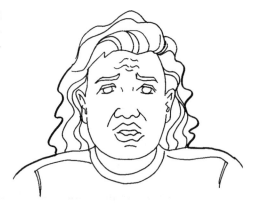

FEAR

Anger n. *Emotional excitement brought on by a strong feeling of displeasure.*

When we are angry, our fists clench, eyes squint, lips squeeze together, and jaws tighten; and our bodies tend to stand still.

I began with the intense emotions of fear and anger because, even though they can be considered negative, the intensity of fear and anger are easy for all of us to understand—as we have surely experienced them at some time in our lives. But, in hearing society, it is socially unacceptable to show these emotions in a physically expressive manner. We are taught to use our tone of voice to convey the message of discomfort or displeasure. In ASL, tone is accomplished through intensity of gesture, facial expression, and movement. The larger the gesture, the more intense the feeling; the smaller the gesture, the more subtle the feeling. Let your body follow its natural inclination to respond; allow yourself to begin to feel a bit out of control. Have fun with it.

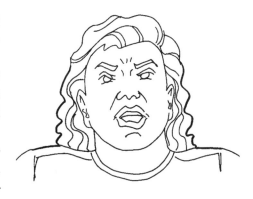

ANGER

Surprise n. *An unexpected gift or event.* v. *To astound or astonish with unexpected wonder or amazement.*

Surprise can be a happy, light feeling. Imagine a time in your life when you experienced a pleasant surprise. Perhaps you were surprised with a special gift or embarrassed by a surprise birthday party. When we are surprised, our eyes and mouths open wide, our hands move upward (palms facing up), and perhaps we even touch our faces. We may step forward, and the upper body leans in the direction of the surprise.

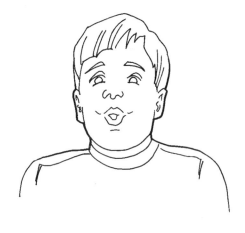

SURPRISE

Shock n. *A source of great emotional disturbance.* v. *To affect with surprise, terror, etc.*

Shock is an intense, extreme emotion. When we feel shock, our hands usually stay near our sides, palms facing downward, and our feet are planted solidly on the floor. The mouth opens wide, while the eyes feel like they want to leap from their sockets. Most of our facial muscles tighten. For this one, you'll really want to see yourself in the mirror!

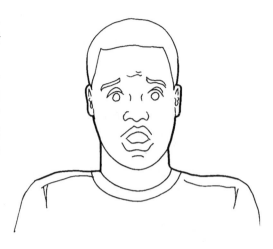

SHOCK

Happiness n. *A pleasant feeling of well-being and/or contentment.*

Really think about something or someone who makes you deliriously happy. Happiness makes the face feel like it is shining: Our eyes glow and our lips almost touch our ears because of our bright, open-mouth smiles. Our hands tend to draw into the body as if we planned to hug ourselves. Go ahead! You are happy!

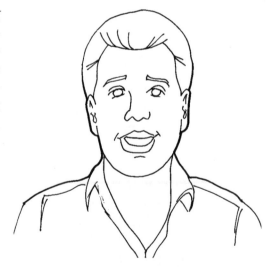

HAPPINESS

Sadness n. *A deep feeling of un-happiness, grief, or depression.*

When you recall a sad experi-ence, and truly feel it, you will immediately become aware of your body's reaction—the oppo-site of how you reacted when you experienced happiness. When sad, our smiles turn into frowns, our hands tend to move down-ward, our eyes droop, and our upper bodies tend to feel heavy. Perhaps the shoulders move downward while the chin wants to touch the chest.

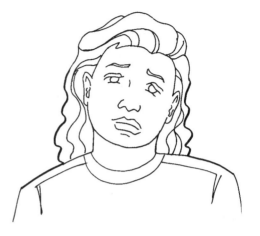

SADNESS

Tiredness n. *Extreme fatigue or lethargy.*

When we feel tired, our shoulders slide into our arms in a long shrug. Our lips pucker into a sigh, and our eyes can barely stay open.

This practice of emotions has made you tired! Now is a good time to pause and take a deep breath. After a short break, continue on to the re-maining emotions on the list.

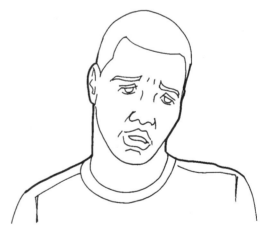

TIREDNESS

Frustration n. *An unsettling feeling of disappointment or dissatisfaction.*

By now, you may have actually experienced this feeling—frustration—while exploring your body's natural expression of emotions. How do our bodies show this frustration? We may feel like we're running but can't reach the finish line. Our chins want to tilt back, and our eyebrows are knitted. We want to throw our hands into the air; with our palms facing forward.

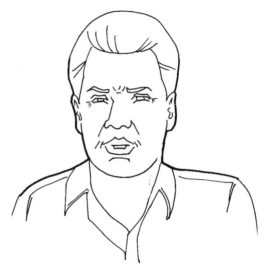

FRUSTRATION

Amusement n. *A pleasant feeling of being entertained.*

Now, it is time to go right ahead and laugh. Release your tension and frustration and feel amused! When amused, the head moves back while the jaws move back and forth as we release air from the back of our throats.

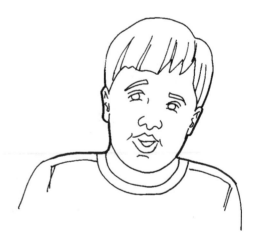

AMUSEMENT

Excitement n. *A strong feeling of arousal to activity.*

Let's get excited about learning ASL! Again, we will feel ourselves smile, while our heels lift from the floor and our hands move to the upper body. Our feet and hands may even feel like dancing!

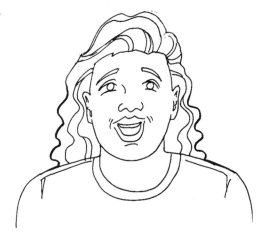

EXCITEMENT

Communicating Emotions with Formal ASL Signs

Hold that feeling of excitement while you study the formal ASL signs for each of the emotions on our list. You will be most pleased to discover how closely the formal signs match the nonverbal, natural movements you have just practiced. Remember, ASL is a three-dimensional language, but the illustrations appear in two dimensions. By practicing the detailed, easy-to-follow instructions, you will learn to properly form and understand the formal signs for our ten emotions.

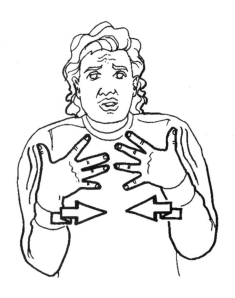

FEAR. Take both hands and open them, extending your fingers. Now, with palms facing your body and the fingers of your left hand facing those of your right hand, move both hands toward each other in front of your chest in one motion. Your fingers do not touch. Remember to lean your shoulders back slightly and use your face to show a fearful expression.

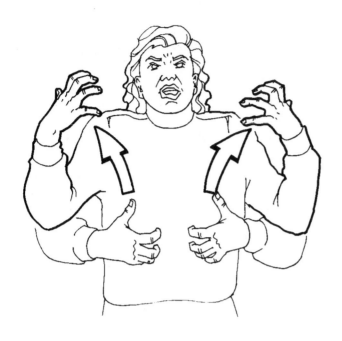

ANGER. The most common sign for anger is one hand (preferably your dominant, or writing, hand) in front of your face with the palm facing in and your fingers crooked like a claw. The use of two hands, as illustrated, adds intensity to the meaning.

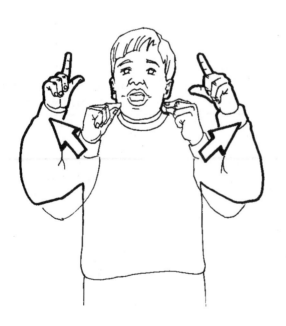

SURPRISE. Assuming you like the surprise, feel your facial expression. Your eyes open wide . . . okay. Take both hands and make fists in front of your lips with the thumbs facing but not touching your eyes. Open your pointer fingers and thumbs wide to form a "C." This shows your "wide eyes" at feeling surprised.

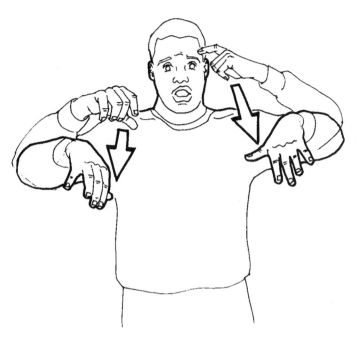

SHOCK. Technically, you can use the same sign as "surprise" but change the facial expression to show shock. Shock and surprise are sometimes closely related in feeling. There is another sign that more precisely fits the direct meaning of *shock*. Point to your forehead with your dominant hand. Then, place both hands in a "C" or "claw" position in front of your chest, elbows bent. Palms face the floor. This sign literally means "mind-numb," the experience of shock.

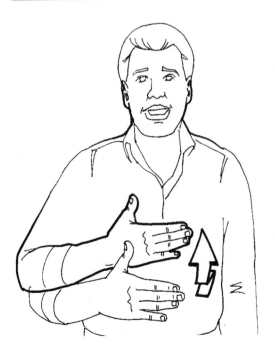

HAPPINESS. Face the palm of your dominant hand toward your body. Place your palm on your chest and move it upward repeatedly, touching your chest. You can use both hands to emphasize a strong feeling of elation. Allow your happiness to show in your posture and facial expression.

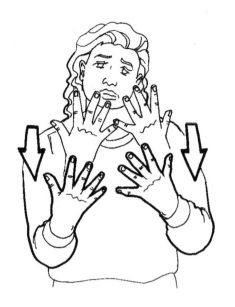

SADNESS. We all know the long face we make when we are sad. The sign for "sad" actually seems to pull the face down even longer. Pull both of your hands down from your eyes (without touching), keeping your fingers spread, palms facing in, and thumbs out. You can be very sad by intensifying your facial expression and making the sign very slowly.

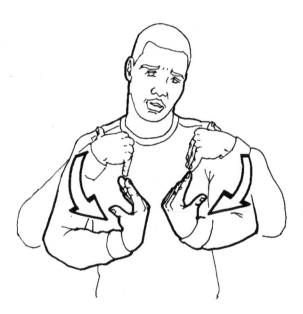

TIREDNESS. Face the palm of your left hand toward your body and place your fingertips on your upper chest, fingers touching the chest and thumb facing toward the ceiling. The wrist is bent to allow for this position. Do the same with the right hand on the right side of your chest. Now, moving both hands at the same time, drop your elbows, allowing the wrists and arms to fall down while your fingers touch your chest. Naturally, you will feel your shoulders drop and you may even breathe a sigh.

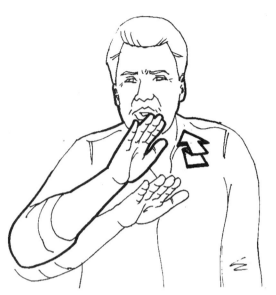

FRUSTRATION. The expression *face a brick wall* illustrates the concept of the formal sign for "frustration." Move the back of your dominant hand under your chin so the backs of your fingers touch your nose. Knit your brows.

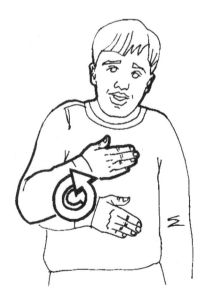

AMUSEMENT. Using your dominant hand, palm facing the body and fingers together, rub your chest repeatedly in a circular motion, which indicates pleasure.

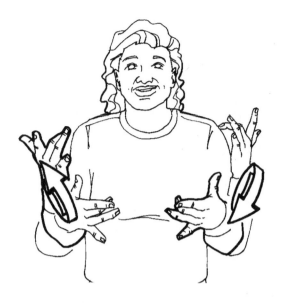

EXCITEMENT. With palms facing your chest, spread your fingers. Bend the middle fingers toward your chest to touch your upper chest. Now, move the middle fingers in an upward motion, still touching the chest. Alternate the movement quickly, first right, then left. Your facial expression and how fast you move your hands will show different degrees of excitement.

EXERCISES

At the end of each chapter, you will find practice exercises, games, or dialogues to make learning ASL even more fun. These exercises are designed to be played in a group or individually. They can be played in a formal classroom, at home with friends or family, or anywhere you feel comfortable.

Emotion Charades

1. Write each of the ten emotions from our list on individual index cards. You may want to make more than ten cards by adding other emotions or feelings to the list. Here are some to try:

• Thirsty	• Guilty	• Confused	• Proud
• Love	• Pain	• Upset	• Sick
• Worry	• Hate	• Innocent	• Hungry
• Dizzy	• Ashamed	• Joy	• Arrogant

Descriptions of the formal signs for these emotions and feelings are listed under "Additional Vocabulary," on page 16.

2. Give one card to each member of the group. Be sure only the person holding the card sees it.

3. Each person should remember the emotion written on his or her card.

4. Collect and shuffle the cards. Place all the cards face up on a table or the floor. The players should stand in a circle around the cards.

5. Anyone can start. The idea is that the players take turns demonstrating the emotion written on their cards. Use the natural body gestures learned in the first part of this chapter. The formal signs may be practiced after the game.

6. After the first person demonstrates their emotion, anyone in the group who recognizes it may step forward and pick up the card for that emotion. The card is shown to the demonstrator. If the card is correct, the demonstrator should nod. No voicing, please! If the card is not correct, the demonstrator should shake their head. Other players may begin to pick up cards until the emotion has been correctly identified.

7. The person who held up the correct card becomes the next demonstrator and shows the emotion written on the card they received at the beginning of the game. Continue taking turns until all of the cards have been identified.

8. Now, you may individually, or in a group, practice the formal signs for these emotions and feelings.

Emotion Charades is a great icebreaker for a beginning sign language class. Students quickly learn a vocabulary of over twenty emotions while establishing the basic skills to fluency in ASL, discovering each of its five essential components. Using body language, feeling, watching, gesturing, employing facial expressions, and having a sense of the space near and around the body are integral to understanding American Sign Language.

Silent Movie

We've all seen silent movie actors and laughed at their use of what now seem to be elaborate gestures to get the characters' feelings across to movie-goers. In this exercise, players must act out an emotional drama for the audience to identify.

1. All players write a sentence on a card that could be a dramatic line of dialogue between two people in a movie. For example, "'Nell, the Mounties will never save you,' said the dastardly villain."

2. The cards are collected, shuffled, and placed in a pile. Players choose partners and each pair chooses a card from the deck.

3. A random audience member reads the line of dialogue on the card aloud while the players must react with the emotions evoked by the words.

4. Audience members call out the emotions successfully portrayed by the actors.

5. Play continues until each pair has given two grand performances!

In the next chapter, we will go one step beyond the simple expression and identification of emotions to explore the big picture painted by natural gesture. Anyone can use natural gesture to describe situations or events, ask questions, tell stories, and more. In fact, without knowing it, we all make use of natural gesture every day—when we look at our watch to say it is time to go and when we raise a hand to hail a taxi. Natural gesture forms the basis of the way in which words or concepts are put together in American Sign Language to make phrases, clauses, and sentences; that is, natural gesture informs the syntax of ASL. Let's take a look at the big picture.

Additional Vocabulary

ARROGANT. Oh, what a fun sign this is! You have heard the expression "a swelled head." Well, that is the concept for this sign. Using your index finger and thumb, form a "C." Your other fingers remain in a fist.

With both left and right hands making the shape, place your left hand on the left side of your head (fingers and thumb pointing toward your scalp). Do the same with the right hand on the right side of your head. Imagine you are placing a crown or halo on your head as you move your hands (still with crooked thumb and index finger) away from your head, as if your head had swollen with an inflated ego. The farther away you move your hands, the "bigger" you represent the arrogant person's head to be.

CONFUSED. This sign uses the "C" or "claw" handshape. To show you are confused, first point to your forehead with your dominant hand. Then, place both hands in the "claw" position with one hand palm facing upward and the other hand palm facing downward, the palms of both hands face each other. Move each hand in a circular motion. Be sure to knit your brows to complete the sign.

DIZZY. Using your dominant hand, curve all your fingers and thumb to form a "C" or "claw" handshape. Since we generally feel dizziness in the area of our heads, this sign is made by moving the "C" or "claw" handshape in front of your face, rotating it in a circular motion, palm facing your face. Remember to include the natural facial expression associated with feeling dizzy (unless, of course, you *are* feeling dizzy—in which case your expression already says it all!).

GUILTY. Make a fist with your right hand. Extend your thumb and index finger to the left. Place this symbol (it also represents the letter "G") on your left upper chest. This sign is formed with your right hand whether you are right- or left-handed.

HATE. Using both hands, touch the middle finger of each hand to its thumb. Now, with palms facing downward and fingers pointing outward, flick your middle finger from your thumb, still pointing away from your body. Imagine you have a sticky piece of lint you are trying to get off of your fingers. Also, remember that when you strongly dislike something, you want to push it away.

HUNGRY. Using your dominant hand, curve all your fingers and thumb to form a "C." Take the "C" hand and touch fingertips and thumb to chest. (This means, of course, your palm is facing your chest.) Now, keeping this handshape, move your hand down the middle of your chest once and stop before you reach your stomach. This sign represents food traveling down your esophagus toward your stomach.

INNOCENT. As always, facial expression is important for this sign. Imagine someone has blamed you for something you did not do. The facial expression you naturally show and feel is the correct one! Now, make fists with both hands. Bring your left fist, palm facing inward, to your left cheek without touching. Bring your right fist, palm facing inward, to your right cheek. Extend the index and middle fingers of both hands toward your lips and move both hands forward away from your face.

JOY. See "happiness" on page 11. "Joy" and "happiness" use the same handshape and movement. To show joy, make your sign more emphatically, as "joy" is a more intense emotion. Let your face show how joyful you are!

LOVE. The word *love* is rich with meaning. There are different signs to express the many connotations of love.

1. The most general sign for "love" is to make a fist with both hands and cross your arms over your chest forming an "X" over your heart.
2. For an even deeper meaning, such as "cherish" or "care," put the palm of your dominant hand under your chin and bring your fingers and thumb down into a fist that touches your chin.
3. The universal sign for "I love you" is also used for greetings and good-byes. It has become so popular, you may have seen the design used for necklaces, pins, keyrings, and other jewelry. Use one hand or for emphasis, both. Extend your index finger and thumb forming an "L." Keeping these fingers extended, lift your little finger. Your middle finger and ring finger are touching your palm. Now, with the "I" (little finger) and "L" (thumb and index finger) still extended, direct the sign toward the person you love, palm facing them and the back of your hand facing you. (Note: The thumb and little finger, when extended, form the signed letter "Y." Hence, this handshape represents "ILY," meaning, of course, "I love you.")

PAIN. Imagine feeling a sharp pain. Take the index finger of your right hand and the index finger of your left hand and point them toward each other, moving them sharply to show pain. You can show how severe this pain is by your facial expression. The sign can be made directly over the part of the body where you are feeling the pain. This is particularly helpful for health care professionals. For example, if you have a headache, form the sign for pain with index fingers pointing toward each other in front of your forehead. If you have a pain in your neck, form the sign in front of the part of the neck that hurts. (Note: This is also the sign for the figurative expression "pain in the neck." You indicate the difference between the literal and figurative meanings by context and facial expression.)

PRIDE/PROUD. Make a fist with your dominant hand. Keeping the fist, take your thumb and move it on your middle chest from your stomach up toward your neck. Think of "Casey at the Bat" and the button that popped from his uniform shirt as his chest swelled up with pride!

SHAME/ASHAMED. You know that old expression "hang your head in shame." Well, that's how you sign it, too. Your head—chin and eyes down—moves to one side. You may add your hand in a cupped position: With the fingers together, cup your hand and turn the palm toward and away from the face so that the back of the fingers touch your cheek, palm facing out, fingers pointed upward. This may feel a bit awkward at first. Be sure you turn your head away from your hand, not into it.

SICK. With palms facing toward your body, spread your fingers straight up and bend the middle finger of each hand toward yourself. Touch one middle finger to your head and one to your stomach. You can feel this sign, as we tend to feel sickness in our heads and stomachs most often.

THIRSTY. Remember how your throat feels dry when you are thirsty? Even your lips tend to pucker. Well, that's the sign: Simply add the index finger (palm facing in) of your dominant hand tracing your throat from chin to Adam's apple one time.

UPSET. Taking your dominant hand, use your index and middle fingers to make a "V." Then take the "V" and turn it, moving downward, several times in front of your stomach. During the motion, your index finger should touch your chest and your middle finger, your stomach.

WORRY. Using both hands, point the fingers upward with thumbs pointing toward your face. Move your hands in a circular motion in front of your face. One hand will move down as the other moves up. Imagine troubled waters as your expression conveys deep concern.

Chapter 2

The Big Picture:
Using Natural Gesture

We see American Sign Language (ASL). As we have already learned, eye contact is the most important component of ASL. As hearing people, we are used to using English words, our ears, and our vocal chords to communicate. By the same standard, ASL is a language people see with their eyes and speak with their bodies, faces, and hands. Remember, words are merely symbols, units of language used to convey meaning. It is how we use these words that produces language and mutual understanding.

ASL Paints Pictures

Visual communication depends on pictures. ASL is a language that paints pictures. Just as spoken and written English depends on an alphabet of letters and sounds, ASL's alphabet depends on movement and expression. *Words*, then, belong to the English language, and *pictures* belong to sign.

Allow your mind to let go of English words. It may be surprising to realize how heavily we rely on words—not only to communicate with others but to think and to process our own thoughts and feelings. In fact, our minds are always drawing on words as an internal method of understanding information. We are always talking to ourselves. Leave the words behind. Just as you did when practicing emotions in Chapter 1, ignore the words to notice the way things look and recognize how you feel about them. To capture the essence of thinking in pictures, which is different from thinking in English words, we must begin to *feel* our way through the process of visualization.

Okay. Take a deep breath. While slowly breathing out, go ahead and call to mind a situation or place that makes you happy. You may conjure a favorite vacation spot, holiday party, or comforting place that is all your own (such as your bedroom, kitchen, playroom, or study). Try to visualize and feel the place, event, or special setting you have chosen. Concentrate on the *picture* and the *feeling* in your mind. Avoid any urge to use words to think about this image or to name any part of it. You may feel uncomfortable at first. That's all right. You're not used to thinking without words.

To feel comfortable enough to begin to learn to communicate in ASL, signers need to enter the *seeing mode*, or characteristic manner of expression, of this beautiful feeling language. Beginning to learn sign language requires you to focus on what things look and feel like rather than what they are called in English. In doing so, you begin to think by using the tools of nonverbal communication. When you consider it, it becomes perfectly natural to think of Deaf people as bilingual—for ASL and English are really two very different languages!

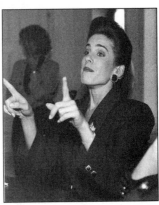

We use natural gestures every day. Here, Heather Whitestone, Miss America 1995, signs "but." Notice the sign is made by moving the fingers away from each other: Wait a minute; hold on!

The Mind's Eye

Practice thinking in images by replacing the English *words* below with *pictures* that describe through your mind's eye:

- Your best friend
- Your favorite sport
- The clothes in your closet
- Sunrise or sunset
- Animals
- A rock concert
- Your house or car
- Going shopping
- Planting a flower garden
- Taking an airplane trip

As the words fall away, allow yourself spontaneously to call to mind whatever images bring the most detail or expressiveness to your pictures. *Feel* each one in turn; *without words*, experience the power your picture conveys in a second's thought!

Now, you will discover how to take the pictures you are holding in your mind and use natural gestures, ASL's building blocks, to paint them in sign. Stand in front of a mirror. Return to the list and choose a

How would you clap without making a sound? Audience members at the Deaf Way Conference show the performer their appreciation by waving their hands in the air.

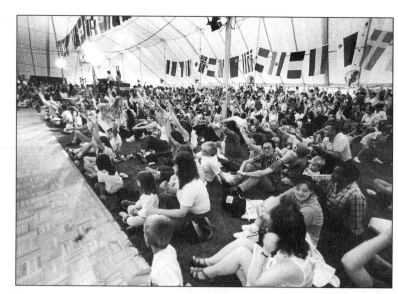

gesture or series of gestures that convey each item. Does spiraling a finger in your hair for "curls" identify your best friend? Does playing air guitar show a rock concert? Does spreading your outstretched arms and fingers in a wide arc over your head paint a sunrise? Does miming hands on a steering wheel mean "driving" or "car"? Quickly, you see the wealth of diverse natural gestures you can choose from to make your mind's pictures come alive and how the same gesture may have more than one meaning or denote different parts of speech, depending on context and use.

The Yellow Room in the House: ASL Grammar Basics

Suppose you want to describe to someone "the yellow room in the house." See your mind's picture. Focus on the picture's most important or biggest subject. This will be the first picture, or sign, in your nonverbal sentence describing the yellow room. Of course, that picture must be of the building the room is in, the house, before you actually can describe the yellow room. Without the "house," we wouldn't have enough information to know where the yellow room belonged. And we couldn't "see" the house unless you had already described it. "House," last in written and spoken English, appears first in sign language. In this way, you begin to prioritize the details of the picture for the person you are signing to. What piece of information is the most vital for establishing a context? Which details are most important for conveying a proper sequence of action? You cannot assume safely that the linear syntax of English grammar will translate word for word into the three-dimensional grammar of ASL. To communicate effectively in sign, you must enter a world of pictures wholeheartedly—using gestures, rhythm, motion, and feeling to show to your partner. Very quickly, you will find that the organization of a spoken English sentence must be conveyed differently in ASL.

Getting the Point across with Natural Gesture

Imagine you are in a foreign country and do not speak the language. You may want to "scream" in English because you are frustrated about trying to get your point across. Remember the formal sign for "frustrated"? (see page 13) Instead of facing a brick wall, you will want to *feel* your way through the situation by using facial expressions, hand and mouth movements, and body language—the tools of nonverbal communication. Let's take a look at two common places we'd surely visit on our foreign travels—a restaurant and a bathroom—and see how easy it really is to communicate in the international language of natural gesture.

Restaurant. Suppose you and your traveling companions are thirsty and you have wandered into a restaurant where you would like to order a glass of milk. You need to know if the restaurant is open and whether it serves milk: "Please, we'd like to have a table and order a glass of milk." In the foyer of the restaurant you catch the attention of the maître d'. The first piece of information you must communicate to the maître d' is "table." Somehow, you must show the maître d' that you would like to be served at the restaurant. Perhaps you use your hands to make the shape of a table. Pretend in a pantomime: Take the pointer finger of your dominant hand and draw a large table in the air or move your flat hand, fingers together and palms facing down, to show the smooth rectangular table surface. Spread a tablecloth on the table; perform the motion. Place a centerpiece on it, filled with fresh flowers. See and feel the environment you are creating in natural gesture. Now, sit down at your table. Call over the waitperson with a wave of the hand, exactly as you would in a real restaurant setting. On your face, give the look of "please." Then, you'll want to get across the action of "drinking." Bring a cup to your lips. How do you sign "milk"? Of course! Pantomime milking a cow. The maître d' has now been thoroughly entertained and, with a nod and a smile, directs you into the lovely café with red checkered tablecloths and wildflowers on each table, where you and your traveling companions can relax. While you enjoy a cold glass of fresh milk, see how close your natural gestures are to the formal signs for "table," "flowers," "drink," "glass," and "milk."

TABLE. Place your dominant hand, fingers together and palm facing down, on top of the elbow of your other arm and make a ledge with the two forearms.

FLOWERS. Touch the thumb and four fingers of your dominant hand together to form an O-shape shape. Bring your fingertips to touch your face on each side of your nose, once to the left and once to the right. You are smelling flowers.

DRINK. The thumb of your dominant hand touches your lower lip. Curve your fingers into the "C" or "claw" shape to suggest a glass or cup. Bring your fingers toward your face, as if you were drinking. (See page 95 for an illustration of this sign.)

GLASS/CUP. Perform the sign for "drink" and put your other hand underneath, palm facing up, to form a base. The base hand signifies the noun "glass" or "cup."

MILK. Take one hand in a milking motion, squeezing your fingers into a fist and pulling down as if you had a cow's udder in your hand. Remember, you only use one hand for the sign, not two.

Bathroom. After much walking through the foreign city's national art museum, it is time to find a bathroom to freshen up. One of your traveling companions spots a museum guard in one of the galleries and sends you over to ask the question, "Where is the bathroom?" This presents a definite challenge. Think about it. Where? First, you must look confused. Remember the formal sign for "confused"? (See page 17.) Be sure to knit your brows and glance about the room. Your head moves in different directions. Perhaps you shrug your shoulders. Now, bathroom. You will need to convey "bathroom" in a socially acceptable manner. You could mime washing your hands by rubbing your palms together. Depending on the situation and urgency, you could put pressure on your stomach or cross your legs and jostle back and forth as a child might do. In no time, the museum guard has pointed you toward relief. Here are the formal signs for "where" and "bathroom."

WHERE. Shake the extended pointer finger (index finger) of the dominant hand in the air, moving the wrist from left to right and keeping the index finger pointed up.

BATHROOM. Make a fist with your dominant hand and place the thumb between the index and middle fingers, palm facing outward.

Shake your hand in the air. You are actually shaking the signed letter "T," used here to mean "toilet." Make this sign, accompanied by a quick shrug, a glance around, and a confused facial expression, and you've asked the question, "Where's the bathroom?" Go ahead, shake a "T"!

EXERCISES

The ability to communicate nonverbally through natural gesture makes us better observers of the world around us. We learn to *look* at situations and *feel* the intensity of our daily exchanges with others. In general, our perceptive powers will increase and deepen as we begin to call on more than just the hearing sense to communicate and to understand. Now we are looking, touching, and seeing.

The following exercises encourage beginning signers to learn as they *do*. The best way to get ready to learn ASL is to throw yourself into the world of natural gestures and nonverbal communication. You will be delighted to discover how many of these gestures are truly second nature to us already.

Can You Help Me?

This is an exercise to do with a partner or in a group. Write down the following situations on individual pieces of paper. One person chooses a sentence, which she or he will act out in natural gesture for the other. The receiving person must ascertain what is being communicated and respond appropriately. A large group can watch each pair, if time allows, or break up into pairs and pass situations from group to group. Make up more situations of your own. There is only one rule: no written or verbal communication allowed!

- Where is the train station? airport? taxi stand? bus station?
- My car's battery is dead. Can you give me a jump start?
- Where do you live? How do I get there from here?
- What type of stores are in the local shopping mall?
- I am looking for a job. Can you give me work to do? What kind of work?

- I need to register for classes. Which classes are still open to students?
- Have you seen [name a movie or TV show]? What is your favorite movie or TV show?
- I want to try out for the basketball team. What will I have to do to make the team?
- Tell me what your occupation is. What are your job duties?
- I just finished a good workout at the gym. Do you work out?

Congratulations! You've just had your first conversations in sign.

Toon Time

Let's test your sense of humor. How long will it take to make your partner laugh?

1. Look through your newspaper's comics or through a collection. Choose a comic strip that allows you to use action to convey the punchline. As some comic strip dialogue may be especially challenging, you should choose a comic with several frames so you will have more concepts to show. Believe it or not, single-frame comics, although seemingly easier, tend to be the most difficult to communicate. A strip such as Gary Larson's *Far Side*, for example, may focus on subject matter that relies heavily on verbal communication and so may not be ideal for this exercise. Some good choices would be *Peanuts*, *Garfield*, *Nancy*, *Hi & Lois*, and *Beetle Bailey*.

2. Act out the strip for your partner. You may want to have a large floor space. Use your whole body to portray different characters and their actions. Remember, everything must be told through natural gesture.

Challenge: See if your partner can not only understand the actions and punchline but also guess which comic strip it is. Go for it.

Moving Art Gallery

The challenge here is to paint the most graphic, interesting, and detailed pictures in the air for your partner as you can. Enjoy yourself; you are the artist.

1. Look through books and magazines to find pictures that are rich
    with action and contain many different things. Good sources are art
    and travel books and magazines such as *National Geographic*, *Art
    News*, and *Sports Illustrated*; advertisements in general magazines can
    also show great variety. Cut out a picture that intrigues you.

2. Without showing the picture to your partner, try to describe it. You
    will find you are painting your pictures in space. Remember, the
    most prominent or important subject will need to be shown first.

3. Now describe all the background things and/or activities. Take as
    much time as you need. Remember, no verbal or written communi-
    cation between partners is allowed.

4. Once you finish painting your picture in natural gesture, your part-
    ner may describe to you in English what they have seen. How
    closely does your picture match the original?

I am sure you are finding that, in addition to using your facial expressions and body language, you need to choose handshapes that best
describe the people, places, or things in your picture. For example, a
tree trunk can be shown with hands curved like a "C," palms toward
each other with your little fingers facing the floor. In this way, you can
"paint" the tree trunk. By moving your hands farther apart or closer together, you can show the size of the tree trunk.

Communicating in Sign. Suppose your picture shows people moving
in some way, such as walking or running. Have you discovered the
trick? Use your index and middle fingers pointing down to represent
legs. Then, let your fingers do the walking or running. Maybe some
people in your picture are sitting or kneeling. Simply adjust your fingers to match. A seated person has bent knees, so bend your two fingers
at the knuckles. If a person is kneeling, you may want to use the up-
lifted flat palm of your other hand to represent the stationary flat surface (grass, sidewalk, etc.) on which the person is kneeling. With your
dominant hand, place your bent knuckles, fingers, and nails on your
still palm.

How many more situations can you describe that use these physical
movements?

As we've now experienced firsthand, communicating nonverbally
with natural gestures provides the basis for forming sentences and

starting a conversation with another person. By exploring natural gesture, new signers begin to understand the fundamental grammatical rules of formal ASL signing. Signers must be aware of the context of the situation, who is present, and what space is occupied. A signer needs to determine what must be conveyed to get the message across, which direction the action moves in, and who is involved. Now, with this knowledge, we are ready to explore the basic elements of formal ASL signs and to see how these elements function in determining meaning and nuance when signing in ASL.

Additional Vocabulary

ANIMAL. As living beings, all animals draw life from their breathing. To make the formal sign for "animal," face the palms of both hands, fingers together toward your chest. Touch the fingertips to the chest and bring the backs of the hands toward each other. Keep the elbows stationary; move the hands from the wrists. Bring the hands together two or three times to show the lungs of the animal expanding and contracting.

CLOTHES. Place the fingertips of both hands on your chest, fingers spread and palms facing toward the body. Move the hands down the chest in one motion. For "pants" or "skirt," make the sign lower on the body, about hip level. For "blouse" or "shirt," make the sign for "clothes" and pull on the item with the thumb and index finger. For "long sleeves," run one hand down the arm. For "short sleeves," tap the upper arm with the flat hand, palm facing up (the pinky finger side of the hand touches your arm).

EXERCISE. As a verb to mean "work out," make fists with both hands and raise the arms in the air as if you are lifting barbells. Use the body's natural resistance when performing the motion to show how hard or easy your workout is!

FRIEND. Take the pointer fingers of each hand and crook them. Connect the fingers at the middle joints to form an "X." Flip the hands over to make the "X" again from the other side. You have shown the act of joining in friendship.

HOUSE. The palms of both hands face each other in front of your body, fingers together. Touch the fingertips of the hands to make an A-frame, like the roof of a house. Then return the hands to the parallel position to indicate the sides or walls of the house.

LEARN. Using your nondominant hand, make a flat page with your palm by holding it out face up with the fingers together. With your dominant hand, use all five fingers to "pick up" the information off the page and put it into your head. Bring your fingertips together to touch the palm of your book page as if you are gathering up information, then touch your fingers to your forehead.

To make the sign for "student," perform the sign above for "learn." Then take your hands, fingers together and palms facing each other, and run them down the torso to represent "a person who learns," or a "student."

MOVIE. Place your nondominant hand with the palm facing toward your body, fingers together, thumb facing toward the ceiling. This is the movie screen. Face your dominant hand palm outward with fingers spread. Join the hands together where the meat of one palm touches the meat of the other. Wiggle the fingers of the dominant hand to show light flickering from the movie screen.

MUSIC. Extend the arm of your nondominant hand straight out in front of you with the palm facing your body. Let your dominant hand hover over the outstretched arm with the fingers together and palm facing toward your body. Rock the hand back and forth over the arm in a curving motion—much like a conductor's wand or the act of playing a musical instrument, such as a violin. Move the hand quickly or slowly to show different beats or tempos.

ROOM. Place both hands in front of your body, palms facing each other and thumbs pointing to the ceiling, fingers together, to show two walls of a room. Now, shift the hands across the body, palms facing you, to make the other two walls. The dominant hand represents the wall of the room closest to your body.

STUDENT. See "learn" above.

SUN/SUNRISE/SUNSET. Using the "C" or "claw" handshape with your dominant hand, place the hand up in the air above your head to indicate the "sun." To say "sun," in the sense of "sunshine,"—"I'll get a sunburn from the rays of the sun"—perform the sign for "sun" and close up the fingers to form an O-shape. Open the fingers up as the palm, facing down, moves toward the body. This shows the sun's rays coming down.

To sign "sunrise" or "sunset," set the arm of your nondominant hand in front of you to represent a horizon line. Rest the other arm on top of it. Using the "C" handshape, move your dominant hand in an arc upward from the elbow for "sunrise" and downward below the elbow for "sunset."

TEACH/TEACHER. With both hands, bring your fingertips together to make an O-shape. Touch your fingertips to your temples, palms facing your body, and pull the hands forward. You are taking the information from your head and giving it to others. You are teaching.

To make the sign for "teacher," perform the sign above. Then take your hands, fingers together and palms facing each other, and run them down the torso to represent "a person who teaches," or a "teacher."

3

The Basic Elements of Formal ASL Signs

By now, you've probably guessed that many of the formal signs in American Sign Language (ASL) found their origins in natural gestures. These gestures, which draw their meaning from our culture, our habits, and our perceptions of the world around us, gradually became streamlined over time into an economical set of symbols. The symbols are made from the elements of formal ASL signs and form the basis of this visual language of expression and movement. ASL, then, has evolved into a sophisticated language where gestures have become incorporated into the actual structure of the language, much as syllables form the common roots of many English words. Formal signs, then, are based on the rules of ASL, just as words are made from the rules of English. The formal signs of ASL have four basic elements:

- Handshape
- Palm orientation
- Hand movement
- Placement

A landmark 1991 research study by Laura Ann Petitto and Paula F. Marentette, cognitive psychologists at McGill University in Montreal, shows that Deaf babies babble with their hands in the same way that hearing babies babble with their voices. The process of learning language is the same for both. As hearing babies begin to make up nonsense words and string sounds together, Deaf babies make up nonsense signs by repeating common handshapes and motions. The scientists discovered that babbling is really the expression of the abstract linguistic structure of any language and allows for the process of absorbing many types of signals, signed or spoken.

As you learn about the four elements of formal ASL signs, what they mean and how they are used, you will see that formal signs are only the starting point for communicating in sign. In the same way that changing a prefix or suffix can affect the meaning of an English word, different elements of formal signs also enhance, enrich, and alter meaning in ASL. Let's see how.

Handshape. Learning to tell the difference between handshapes is important to understanding meaning. The formal signs we have learned in previous chapters use many handshapes, including the "C" or "claw," the pointing finger, the O-shape, the fist, and the flat five-hand (with fingers together or spread apart). We know that handshapes used in different ways mean different things, the same way similar sounds can be put together in many combinations to form various English words. Handshapes, like sounds, are morphemes: minimal grammatical units of a language, each constituting a word or a meaningful part of a word that cannot be divided into smaller meaningful parts.

When you keep the same handshape but change any one or more of the other basic elements—palm orientation, hand movement, or placement—the *meaning changes*. Study the illustrations of the formal signs for "yours," "ours," and "mine."

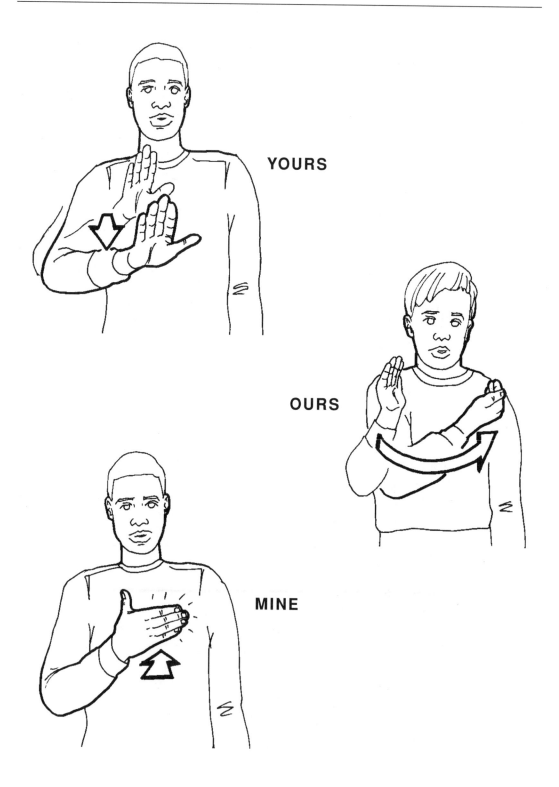

YOURS

OURS

MINE

For "yours," the palm orientation, hand movement, and placement are all *away* from the speaker and toward the other person: "It is yours." For "ours," the palm orientation, hand movement, and placement are circular to encompass both the speaker and his or her companions: "It is ours." For "mine," the palm orientation, hand movement, and placement are all toward the speaker: "It is mine." All three signs use the flat five-hand handshape.

Fluent ASL signers can build beautiful lyrical paragraphs without ever changing handshape but by simply changing one or more of the other basic elements of the signs. Now, we can see the fluidity and grace of ASL. Signing well does not mean making the best literal word-for-word translation from spoken English but choosing the most articulate and beautiful signs to enhance meaning. Like a poet uses rhyme, hard and soft consonants, punctuation, alliteration, and other linguistic devices to evoke emotion and add dimension to written and spoken English, fluent signers use the basic elements of signs, along with body language and facial expressions, to create beautiful expressions in ASL.

Palm Orientation. Palm orientation can be possessive, as we saw in the formal signs for "yours," "ours," and "mine," depending on where the palm is facing. Palms facing toward your body or upward are generally elements of a positive sign; palms facing downward or away from the body usually indicate negatives. We can see how palm orientation, a structural element of the linguistics of ASL, traces back to natural gesture.

Let's take a look at what we "know" and "don't know."

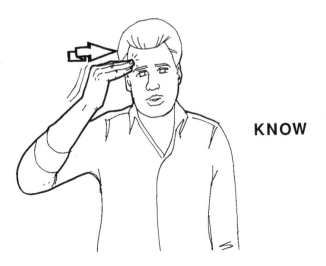

KNOW

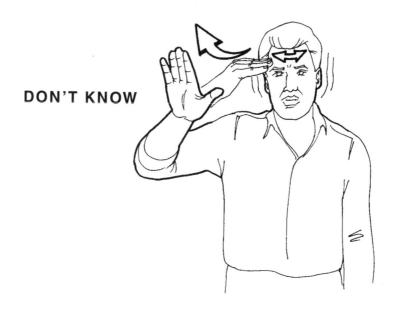

DON'T KNOW

Both formal signs use the five-hand handshape. When the palm, facing inward toward the body, moves close to touch the head and the forehead at the temple, it means "know": "I possess the knowledge." When the inward-facing palm moves across the forehead and then away from the body—literally pushing the palm out as in the sign for "yours," it means "don't know." The head shakes no simultaneously: "I do not possess the knowledge." The change in palm orientation is crucial to understanding the difference in the meaning of the two signs.

As hearing people, we learn to do more than simply imitate signs, but to feel them. In this way, we become more sensitive to both the receptive and expressive aspects of ASL. Practice the signs for "know," "don't know," "yours," "ours," and "mine," in front of a mirror. Focus on performing the signs correctly and on the proper facial expressions, mouth movements, and body language appropriate to each. Allow what you have learned about natural gesture to enhance the meaning of each sign you make. Consider the emotional content of these signs as well.

GOOD. With the dominant hand, take the five-hand with fingers together and the palm oriented toward the body. Touch the fingertips to your mouth and move the hand down in an outward motion so that the palm faces up; your wrist remains stationary. Use your other hand as a base to receive it, palm also facing up.

BAD. Begin to perform the sign for "good." This time, after your fingertips touch your mouth, push the palm away from the body face down.

Hand Movement. How the hand moves when performing a sign provides further nuances in meaning. Hand movements can even function as a descriptor of the sign itself. Broad movements could mean large or open, while restricted movements could mean small or tight. Signs made quickly or slowly can convey a rush or no hurry. If a sign is made in a repetitive motion, performing the sign over and over, it connotes repeated action. But if a sign is made in a circular motion, it connotes continual action. For example, the sign for "work."

WORK. The sign for the verb "work" is the same as the sign for the noun "job." Make fists with both hands. Place your dominant fist, wrist down, on top of the wrist of your other hand. Gently move the dominant hand up and down, touching at the wrists with palms facing down. Striking the fists together three or four times means "I worked and worked; I worked a lot." Performing the sign over and over again means "a lot." If you strike the wrists together once and then move them together in a clockwise circular motion, you never stopped working at any time.

Now look at the sign for "depend."

DEPEND. The extended pointer (or index) finger of the dominant hand touches the nail of the pointer finger of the other hand and presses it down. You can use this sign to mean "it depends," in answer to a question such as "Are we going to go to Gallaudet tonight or tomorrow?" The same sign can have a verb usage, as in "I depend on you to learn sign language well." For both of these uses, the formal sign is performed once.

If you perform the sign for "depend" in a continual circular motion, pushing the circle out toward its object, "you," it means "I am dependent upon you." You have illustrated the state of dependency.

Placement. Formal signs located close to the body usually indicate the signer, while those located away from the body indicate something or someone the signer is referring to. Placement, or location, is often used to establish pronouns (you, me, us, she, he, it) or noun subjects in conversation.

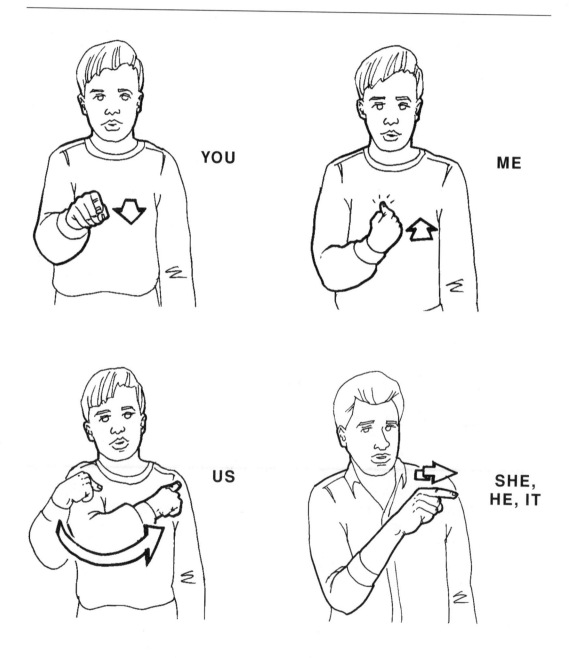

YOU

ME

US

SHE,
HE, IT

Note that the handshape for each pronoun is the extended pointer finger of the dominant hand. Pronouns can be expressed by pointing to the appropriate person, if that person is in the room. In hearing society, it is considered impolite to point in public, but in the Deaf community it is an accepted and important way to communicate quickly and efficiently. In ASL, pointing is an integral part of the grammatical and syntactic structure of sign and is used for many purposes. For example, for an object that is the central subject of discussion—the house or the table—it would be proper to perform the formal sign for the object the first time it is mentioned in conversation and then point to it; so, "table," point. Thereafter, you can simply point to the object during the conversation without again repeating the sign, because you have established that you are discussing the table.

Now, suppose you are telling your sister or brother about what happened in school today. You want to tell a story about two classmates. Remember the formal sign for "student" from Chapter 2 (on page 30)? By performing the sign for "student" and pointing to the left, you are establishing, "There's Student #1." By performing the sign and pointing to the right, you are establishing "There's Student #2." Neither student, of course, has come home with you; only you and your sibling are in the living room. From now on, as you tell your story, you will point to the left for Student #1 and to the right for Student #2. You have used three dimensions to establish pronoun references in your conversation.

Point to left = Student #1
Point to right = Student #2

When "Student #1 said," you turn your head and eyes to the left and point to that spot. When "Student #2 did," you turn your head and eyes to the right and point to that spot. In your conversation, the points in the air represent the students. This can be confusing for beginning signers to follow, because you must remember every point that is established and who that point signifies. Within the Deaf community, pointing usually isn't even necessary; a nod or glance to the correct spot is enough to get to the point!

EXERCISES

By now, you've discovered that by using the elements of the formal ASL signs (handshape, palm orientation, hand movement, and placement) you can make numerous signs and convey a great deal of information with speed and accuracy. These exercises will hone your skills at recognizing and using the four basic elements that are so important to communicating in ASL.

It's All in the Hands

How many formal signs can you make from one handshape? "Think" about it!

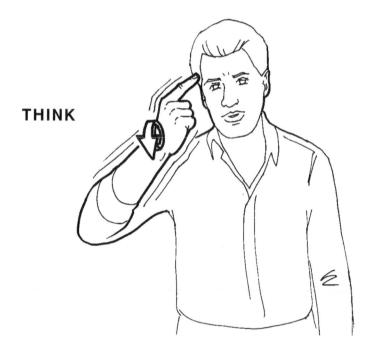

THINK

Using the pointer finger handshape, you've learned to sign many things: "you," "me," "us," "she/he/it," "I," "think," "where," "friend," and "thirsty. " In a group, or on your own in front of a mirror, see how many formal signs or natural gesture signs you can make using each of the following handshapes. Use only one handshape at a time.

- Pointer finger
- "C" or "claw" handshape
- Five-hand, fingers together or spread apart
- Fist
- O-shape

ASL poets compose beautiful verse-sign that concentrates on the lyrical movement of one fluid handshape.

Story Hands

This is an exercise to do in a group. Choose one handshape from the list in the previous exercise. Sitting in a circle, one group member begins a story by making a formal or a natural gesture sign using that handshape. The next person in the circle must contribute a sign to continue the story. How long can you keep your story going? Tell a new story for each of the five handshapes.

Here are two story strings to get you started:

1. I think you . . .
2. My room in the house . . .

Challenge: While using one handshape, change the elements of formal ASL signs—palm orientation, hand movement, and placement—to continue your story. How many details can you add? Remember facial expressions and body movements! Have fun with it.

So far, we've learned a lot about how to see and think with natural gesture. We've studied the basic elements of formal signs and some of the rules that make up the grammar and syntax of formal signing in ASL. You are gaining confidence in expressing yourself more comfortably with your facial expressions, body movements, and hand movements. Now you are eager to take what you've learned and use it to communicate in sign with others. Perhaps you are ready to ask a Deaf coworker, friend, or relative to spend time with you to practice or fine-tune your new skills. In the next chapter, we will enter the world of the Deaf community to gain insight into ASL's natural signers, find out more about the Deaf culture, and discover the particular concerns and challenges of being Deaf in a society that has a hearing majority.

ADDITIONAL VOCABULARY

GO. Hold both hands in front of your body with the pointer fingers extended up toward the ceiling. Move the fingers at the same time in an arc to point out away from you. This is the same sort of motion that ground control personnel at airports use to wave an airplane toward the gate. You can use this sign to show the direction something is going in, by pointing appropriately in context.

FOLLOW. Make fists with both hands and point the thumbs up toward the ceiling. Touch knuckles of the nondominant hand against the base of the thumb of the dominant hand. Move both hands forward, away from the body. The nondominant hand "follows" the dominant one.

MEET/MEETING. Hold both hands in front of your body with the pointer fingers extended up toward the ceiling. Palms face each other. Move the hands together so that the bases of the palms meet.

For "meeting," perform the sign for "meet" with all the fingers (not just the pointer finger) extended upward. Bring only the fingertips together to touch, representing a group of people getting together.

PRACTICE. With the dominant hand, touch your fingertips to the palm, the thumb points to the ceiling, palm facing out. (This is actually the signed letter for "A.") Rub the flat middle section of the A-hand's fingers back and forth over the extended pointer finger of the non-dominant hand. You are "brushing up."

SIGN (IN ASL). Take both fists and place them in front of your chest, palms facing each other. In a circular motion that moves out away from your body, alternately open and close each fist. You are literally throwing concepts into the air.

SLEEP. Using your dominant hand, place the flat five-hand with the fingers spread apart in front of your face, palm facing toward you. Pull the hand down the face while bringing the fingers together and dropping your head. Imagine pulling your eyes closed. You are falling asleep!

STUDY. Using your nondominant hand, make a flat page with your palm by holding it out face up with the fingers together. With your dominant hand, take the flat five-hand with fingers spread apart and bend from the wrist so the fingertips aim down at the page hand. Wiggle the fingers of the dominant hand back and forth to show the eyes studying the page as information is absorbed. (See "learn" on page 30.)

WALK. Using the five-hand handshape, fingers together and palms facing down, bend both hands at the wrist and alternate moving them back and forth to show the motion of walking.

Chapter 4

Deaf Culture

What is the most important thing a hearing person must know about Deaf culture? We've learned that signing and understanding in American Sign Language (ASL) depends, above all, on eye contact. People must be able to see each other to converse in ASL. As you've enjoyed practicing the exercises and vocabulary in this book, you have found yourselves participating in group activities where your attention was focused and directed toward one another. You experienced the exchange of communication flowing from your faces, bodies, hands, and feelings. Perhaps you have begun to recognize and appreciate the immediacy and power of communication, face to face, in ASL. Even when studying on your own, you probably use a mirror to observe your progress and sharpen your skills. If the language of Deaf culture depends on the ability to see, as we know firsthand that it does, then Deaf culture itself must also be visually based.

Seeing the Connection

Suppose your department at work has just hired a Deaf employee whose help you'll need to complete an important project. You approach the open door of the new employee's office and find them diligently concentrating, with their back facing you, on work at the computer. What do you do? How do you get the Deaf person's attention? You can't knock on the door, or quietly say the person's name—the Deaf person cannot hear you. In hearing society, it would be rude to simply walk into someone's office unannounced, much less walk up to a stranger and touch them from behind. Even so, a person who can hear would be able to detect the sounds you make as you walk into their office and would have some time to react and turn around, while a Deaf person cannot hear your approach. Do you walk in anyway and touch the person on the shoulder? Have you come up with the best solution? Of course! Flick the light switch and wait for them to acknowledge you. This easily gets the Deaf person's attention and also allows time for them to react to your presence and get ready to converse with you—*before* you have entered the Deaf person's personal space. Once again, the visual cue is the key to communication.

If you cannot find the light switch, or its location is not convenient, entering the office to tap the Deaf person on the shoulder is acceptable. In Deaf culture, touch becomes an important way to communicate when no visual cue is available. Still, everyone likes to have reaction time. Some Deaf people will put a pocket mirror on their office computers to act as a sort of rear-view mirror. This helps the Deaf person remain aware of movement in the office and prevents them from experiencing the constant annoyance of interruptions from behind that can be commonplace in a work environment.

Has the light come on yet for us? Deaf people share a unique life experience—the perception of the world around them without the sense of hearing. This life experience shapes their beliefs, activities, and interactions, both among themselves and with hearing people. Anthropologists, in their study of the social interactions of humankind, assert that a shared life experience forms the basis for the development of culture and community. As a culture establishes itself, it gives birth to language. ASL is the language of Deaf culture. In this chapter, you will be learning more about Deaf culture and the Deaf experience.

Acceptance of ASL

In 1955 when educator Bill Stokoe came to Gallaudet University to teach English, the university enrolled him in a class to learn how to sign. Stokoe quickly noticed that the signs his own students made seemed far more complex and expressive than the ones he was learning from his classroom teacher. Could ASL be a language? he wondered. Believe it or not, the idea was revolutionary. Linguists at that time believed language was based on speech and sound; ASL's movements in space didn't fit that definition. "What I said," Stokoe explains, "is that language is not mouth stuff—it's brain stuff." Stokoe went on to write the first dictionary of ASL formulated on linguistic rules.

Today, ASL and English are recognized as two *different* languages. ASL is acknowledged as the third most common language in the United States—after English and Spanish. ASL is used by more than half a million Americans. Neurologist and best-selling essayist Oliver Sacks, author of *The Man Who Mistook His Wife for a Hat* and *Seeing Voices*, says ASL is "a language equally suitable for making love or speeches, for flirtation or mathematics."

But there was a time when ASL was forbidden in the education of the Deaf and "oralism," the practice of lipreading English, became the standard for teaching language to Deaf children. Oralism was adopted at the Congress of Milan, an international meeting of educators held in 1880, infamous among Deaf people. Out of several hundred congress attendees, only two were Deaf. The congress announced "the incontestable superiority of speech over sign" and voted to banish ASL. Before the congress, every American school for the Deaf taught in

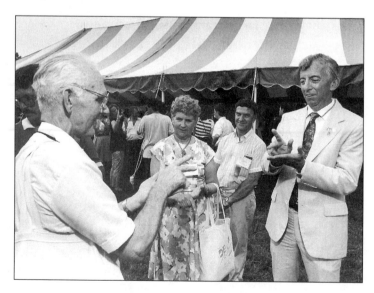

I. King Jordan, president of Gallaudet University (at right), signs to Dr. Gerald Burstein, a Deaf community leader, during festivities at the Deaf Way Conference held in Washington, D.C.

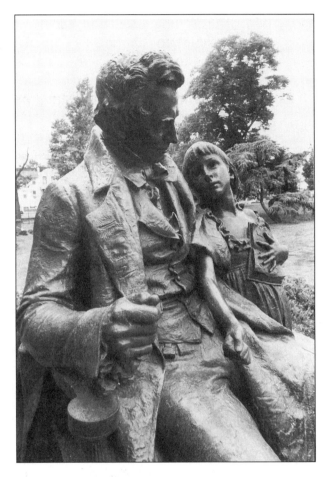

Thomas Hopkins Gallaudet teaches his first pupil, Alice Cogswell, her name in sign language. They are performing the signed letter "A." Gallaudet University was founded in 1864 by his son, Edward Miner Gallaudet; Abraham Lincoln signed the bill that allowed the school to be recognized as a university.

ASL—by 1907, none did. It is hard to believe that the famous inventor of the telephone—the communications-facilitating device that literally changed the world—Alexander Graham Bell, himself married to a Deaf woman, was a staunch oralist. The president of the National Association of the Deaf at the time called the inventor the "most to be feared enemy of the American Deaf." This is how powerful the movement against ASL became.

ASL, however, was cherished and preserved by Deaf families who passed the language down through generations. Students at Deaf residential schools used ASL freely in the dormitories, even though they were reprimanded for using it in the classroom. Where there is a shared experience, there is culture. Within a culture, there is language. Today, educators follow the Bilingual-Bicultural model advanced by Northeastern

University linguist Harlan Lane, author of *The Mask of Benevolence*, an important book about Deaf language and culture. Deaf children are encouraged to learn ASL as their native language and to learn written English as a *second* language. The residential school remains an important place for deaf children of hearing parents to "find out how to be Deaf," as Lane puts it. Deaf people often meet their spouses while at school.

There are more than sixteen million Americans with some degree of hearing loss, but to be a full member of the Deaf community, the deaf person must use ASL and promote its use in schools and its acceptance among hearing people. Championing ASL as a language is very important to Deaf culture.

Common Misconceptions about Deafness

Because they have not been exposed to Deaf culture, or may not have ever met a Deaf person, many people in hearing society harbor several misconceptions about deafness and communicating with Deaf people. These misconceptions often lead to misunderstandings when a Deaf person interacts with a hearing person. Let's take a look at the most common misconceptions some hearing people may have about deafness.

Hearing aids restore hearing and help a Deaf person to understand spoken English.

Hearing aids do no more than amplify sounds. Someone may have a level of hearing loss that permits them to recognize only low voices, or only high ones. A hearing aid will not enable that person to hear what they cannot *already* register—it will simply increase the volume. And hearing aids do not assist a person's ability to discriminate and process sounds; a Deaf person may be able to "hear" environmental noises, such as cars passing by and human voices, but may not be able to discern words. Hearing aids are important tools, however, that allow Deaf people to keep in touch with their environment and provide them with important clues about what is happening in the world around them.

Deaf people can read lips and understand almost everything that is spoken in English.

Nearly all Deaf people read lips at some time, and some are more comfortable with it than others. But regardless of ability or comfort level, studies have shown that Deaf people are able to get only 20 to 30 percent of conversational content when lipreading and can identify perhaps three or four words out of every ten. Most speech in English is made at the back of the throat, not on the lips. Imagine, for instance, trying to tell the difference between "I love you" and "island view" or to distinguish between rhyming and almost-rhyming words like "sit," "knit," "bit," "pit," and "get." Try turning down the volume on your TV set to discover other obstacles to lipreading successfully: The speaker continually puts their hands or hair over the face; the speaker has a mustache or beard; the room is too bright or too dark to see clearly; the speaker turns away, looks down, or leaves the room but continues to speak. Lipreading can be a difficult task. It is fatiguing and inexact, yet some Deaf people, raised in the oralist tradition, still rely on lipreading as a primary means of communication.

It is important to note that there are oral interpreters. Oral interpreting is usually used in a group situation, such as a meeting with many spontaneous speakers, where the Deaf person could not possibly keep up with conversation by reading lips. The oral interpreter is trained to mouth words for the Deaf person to be easily read on the lips and to use clear and precise mouth movements.

Deaf people should learn to speak.

For the profoundly Deaf person, learning to speak when you have never heard sounds is like trying to visualize a place you have never seen before and for which there is no description. Even for those with some hearing, it can still take years to learn the simplest of words. For Heather Whitestone, Miss America 1995, a talented, intelligent young woman with some residual hearing, it took many years of training to be able to speak her last name correctly. That's a lot of time and effort!

While a Deaf person with some hearing may want to use speech, it is important for hearing people to accept that many Deaf people prefer not to speak. While some Deaf people will use speech in their interactions with hearing people, among the Deaf themselves speaking is unnecessary. Speech is associated with hearing society's rejection of ASL, the natural language of Deaf people, and so it is considered unnatural and confining to the Deaf community.

Deaf people use sign language.

Many people with a hearing loss do not use ASL. Some have enough hearing to function successfully through a combination of hearing and lipreading. Some have lost their hearing as a result of getting older, and often such people don't admit to the degree of hearing loss they have experienced. Some, unfortunately, have not been exposed to an environment where sign language can be learned. Most people who become deaf early in life or are born deaf do learn ASL.

Deaf people are not as intelligent as hearing people.

Hearing ability has nothing to do with intelligence. When a Deaf person has problems expressing themselves in written or spoken English, it does not mean that person is not capable of understanding. It could mean that the Deaf person has not developed competency in language skills as far as they could.

Deaf people are all alike.

Deaf people are as diverse in interests, tastes, talents, and viewpoints as the rest of us. Their dreams and goals are equally as limitless—just

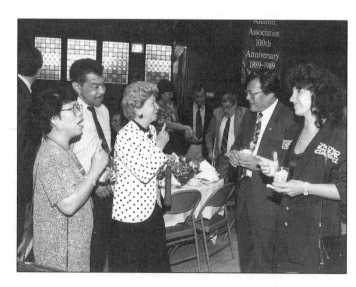

Gallaudet graduates enjoy each other's company and share success stories as they celebrate the Alumni Association's 100th anniversary.

look at accomplished people such as Oscar-winning actress Marlee Matlin; athlete Shelley Beattie of television's *American Gladiators* and a member of the all-female crew of *America³* who competed for the America's Cup; renowned ASL poet Clayton Valli; and educator James Tucker, superintendent of the Maryland School for the Deaf.

Celebrating Deafness

What does it mean to be deaf? Most people in the hearing community would say that being deaf means not being able to hear. Some may be more explicit in categorizing the inability to hear as a "loss"—a person is deprived of the sense of hearing or their hearing has been taken away from them. This viewpoint follows the pathological, or disease model, of deafness. To the Deaf community, the pathological model is brainwashing. Deafness is a reality that shapes Deaf people's life experiences. Deafness is a part of a person's identity to be cherished and nurtured with pride, not dismissed as a tragedy. Deaf people do not want their hearing to be "fixed" so that they can become more like hearing people. A recent survey shows that 86 percent of Deaf adults say they would refuse a cochlear implant, even if it were free.

The Deaf community celebrates Deafness. The birth of a Deaf child to Deaf parents is a joyous occasion. In hearing society, the birth of a deaf child is seen as a grieving event; hearing parents are nervous, worried, and concerned that their child will not grow up to be "normal," that is, hearing. But for the Deaf, the birth of a deaf child *is* normal and exciting—the deaf child will grow up to use their visual language, ASL, and become fluent in both ASL and written English. The child will participate in and preserve Deaf culture. To hearing parents of deaf children who may be turning to this book for guidance, the message of the Deaf community is clear: Though it may be hard to give up the hearing identity you envisioned for your child, there is a great gift you can give to your deaf child. Accept the child's identity as a Deaf person, accept ASL as the child's first language and learn the child's natural language with them, be welcomed with your child into the Deaf community, which will support and nurture your family's identity. Instead of mourning, celebrate! Strengthen the child's self-esteem and share in their culture.

The illustrator of this book, Paul Setzer, is a Deaf adult whose parents are hearing. He is married to a Deaf woman, whose parents are also hearing, and they have five bright, wonderful children. After a meeting to talk about the illustrations for this book, Paul's wife showed us pictures of the children and pointed them out—Deaf, Deaf, Deaf, hearing, Deaf. "Hearing?" we asked. Paul's wife signed, "It just happened." In this family, a *hearing* child was unexpected; but hearing or deaf, the identity of the child is cherished and a Bilingual-Bicultural household is the norm.

Becoming a Member of the Deaf Community

As you continue your study of ASL, undoubtedly you have become greatly curious about Deaf culture and are eager to know more about how to participate in the Deaf community. Here are some ways to improve your sign skills and to get involved in activities that will enable you to use ASL correctly and communicate effectively in the language of the Deaf community:

- Watch videotapes.
- Try to become friends with a Deaf person. Perhaps you have a family member who is Deaf or a coworker. Seek out this person's company and let them know you want to learn about their culture and language.
- Get involved in the Deaf community. Ask a Deaf loved one or friend to invite you to accompany them to Deaf events.
- Go to plays performed by Deaf actors in ASL.
- Join an ASL study group or tutoring program.
- Volunteer in a setting where you will find Deaf people, such as a Deaf residential school.
- Take classes in ASL at your local community college. Seek out Deaf students who may be attending your local college or university.
- Read books about deafness and Deaf culture (see "Suggested Reading" on page 153). Subscribe to Deaf publications.
- Find a buddy to be your partner in sign, to practice ASL with you regularly and exchange face-to-face communication.

Becoming a member of the Deaf community means more than just learning ASL. You must be willing to enter the Deaf experience. After an extensive study of Deaf culture, two linguists at Gallaudet University, Charlotte Baker and Dennis Cokely, developed the following diagram in 1980, which explains how a person qualifies to become a full member of the Deaf community.

Deaf culture is at the core of the diagram. To fully participate and be accepted into Deaf culture you *must* possess each of the four characteristics that define it: audiological, social, political, and linguistic. The Deaf community at large is illustrated by the shaded portions of the diagram. To participate in the Deaf community, you must have at least two of the defining characteristics. Let's examine each one.

Audiological. You must have a hearing loss. It does not matter if you are profoundly deaf (70 decibel loss or higher) or are hard-of-hearing (40 to 60 decibel loss). To a Deaf person, hearing loss means deafness,

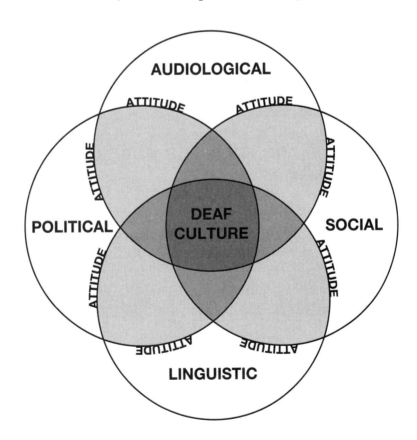

period. *Deaf* is used to describe a life experience rather than denote a degree of hearing loss. In fact, *hearing-impaired* is a term used primarily by hearing society. To a hearing person, *hard-of-hearing* or *hearing-impaired* describes a person who is easier to communicate with than a *deaf* person. Deaf culture does not use qualifying labels for hearing loss. Keep in mind, however, hearing loss alone does not qualify a deaf person for core membership in Deaf culture. A deaf person who is an oralist and who does not support ASL or participate in Deaf social events or politics won't be accepted. The Deaf consider such a person "hearing-minded," and feel they've missed out on the language and beliefs of the Deaf community.

Social. A person must join in the social fabric of the Deaf community. This could mean attendance at a Deaf residential school or having Deaf family members, friends, partners, or spouses. A hearing person who goes regularly to Deaf community events, uses ASL, and advocates Deaf issues—a sign-language interpreter, for instance—will come as close to the core of Deaf culture as a person can who has no actual hearing loss.

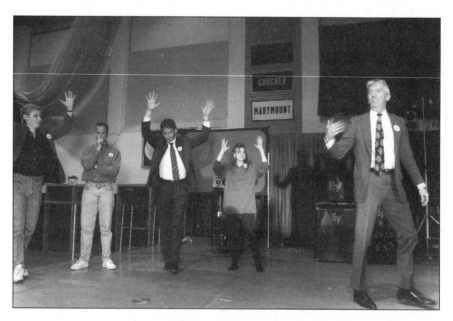

Greg Hlibok, president of the Student Body Government, and other students share the stage with I. King Jordan during the Deaf President Now movement.

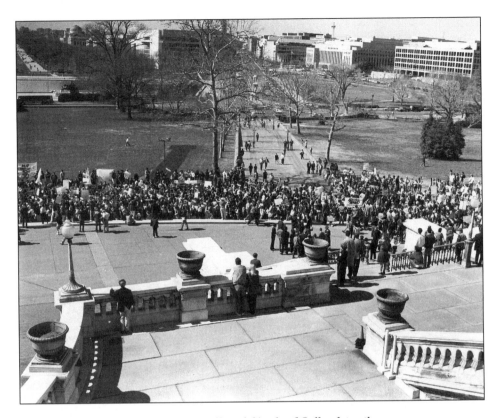

Students, faculty, staff, and friends of Gallaudet gather
at the Deaf President Now rally at the
nation's Capitol Building.

As we know, Deaf culture is visually based. Face-to-face communication, therefore, is considered precious. Frequent meetings with friends and family to socialize and network are necessary to maintain a strong close-knit Deaf community and give Deaf people opportunities to pass along and receive information from one another. Local Deaf clubs flourish, and people come from all over the country to attend Deaf tournaments in sporting events like bowling, chess, and softball. There is even an international Deaf Olympics.

Today, because of advances in technology, Deaf people can communicate more easily from the home than was possible even a decade ago. Telecommunication Devices for the Deaf (TDDs), also called TTYs, make phones accessible to Deaf users, and all states now offer federally mandated Telephone Relay Services where an operator will voice a Deaf person's TTY message to a hearing person on the other end of the line. Faxes, computers, on-line services, and e-mail all make communication swift and manageable from a distance. Closed-captioning allows Deaf people to keep up with broadcast news events and enjoy filmed entertainment. Nothing, however, takes the place of direct human interaction and signing face to face remains the most important and preferred method of communication among the Deaf.

Political. A person must be a passionate advocate of ASL and Deaf issues. Political members of the Deaf community are usually Deaf people with visible positions of authority at an organization like the National Association of the Deaf or a Deaf publication such as *Silent News*. The successful campaign of Gallaudet students in 1988 to have a Deaf president named to the university for the first time in its 126-year existence is considered a major breakthrough for Deaf culture. Dr. I. King Jordan was appointed to the presidency and holds the position today.

Linguistic. ASL must be used and advocated. Students of ASL need to do more than memorize and imitate a list of vocabulary, they must learn to make sentences, ask questions, provide information, and carry on a conversation. They must learn and respect the etiquette and customs of Deaf culture and use them to sign properly in ASL. Just as a French person, for example, demands a respect for the native French language and culture before they will accept a foreigner, so does the Deaf community require the same consideration from ASL signers.

Attitude. Each of the characteristics defining the Deaf community are linked by *attitude*. A person must love the Deaf experience. With the proper respect, enthusiastic involvement, and open-minded willingness to learn about deafness and Deaf issues, you will be accepted by the Deaf community—whether you are a hearing person or a deaf person.

As you meet more members of the Deaf community and work to gain acceptance, you may meet a little resistance from some Deaf people. A Deaf person may find you are learning to sign in ASL and may even compliment your progress, but revert to signing in English word order in your presence. Remember that Deaf people are used to accommodating the needs of hearing society and may naturally assume that this is what is necessary. Deaf people must become skilled and proficient at English to succeed in the community at large because our society has a hearing majority. Take the extra time and effort to convince your Deaf friends that you want to learn to make your way in *their* environment—and that means without English!

Practice, practice, practice ASL!

Working with Sign Language Interpreters

The Americans with Disabilities Act (ADA), signed into law by President Bush on July 26, 1990, is facilitating the link between Deaf people and hearing people by mandating a Deaf person's right to appropriate services and technology. We've already mentioned TTYs and closed-captioning. Qualified sign language interpreters also provide an important service. Through an interpreter, a Deaf person can communicate quickly and effectively with a hearing person who has no knowledge of ASL. Interpreters work with Deaf individuals in educational settings, legal settings, health care settings, religious settings, entertainment settings, and business and industry settings. Interpreters facilitate communication for Deaf and hearing consumers—in short, anywhere a Deaf person may go where effective and accurate communication *must* be ensured.

Here's the formal sign for sign language interpreter.

SIGN LANGUAGE INTERPRETER. Bring the thumb and index finger of both hands together with the other fingers extended. This looks like the natural gesture for "okay." Join the thumbs and index fingers together to make a figure eight. Then switch to make the figure eight from the other direction. A link in the chain of communication between Deaf and hearing is forged.

A qualified interpreter is defined by the U.S. government as "an interpreter who is able to interpret effectively, accurately, and impartially both receptively and expressively, using any necessary specialized vocabulary." Sign language interpreters are professionally trained and have the ability to move between English and ASL (and vice versa) with ease. Ideally, interpreters should be certified by the national Registry of Interpreters for the Deaf.

Interpreters act simply and *only* as intermediaries. Always remember to address the Deaf person directly and speak to the Deaf person in the first person. Talking to the interpreter and referring to the Deaf person as "him" or "her" is awkward and embarrassing for everybody. The interpreter's job is to render *all* communication faithfully, in a neutral and impartial manner, and with strict confidentiality. For these reasons, friends and family members of Deaf persons should not be asked to interpret in most situations. Not only could it be difficult emotionally but the loved one might not possess the specialized vocabulary needed in a specific setting.

You can help by advocating for qualified interpreters at your school, in your community, and at your place of business.

Deaf Hearing Understand

By learning ASL, you are a part of the connection between Deaf culture and hearing society. By keeping an open mind and showing a willingness to learn and understand, Deaf and hearing people will be able to share the richness of their combined experiences.

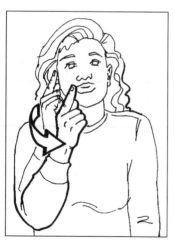
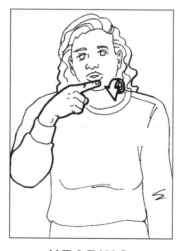
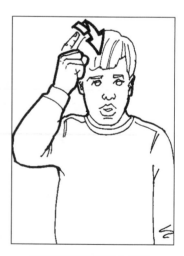

DEAF   **HEARING**   **UNDERSTAND**

So, you are introducing yourself to the new Deaf employee we met at the beginning of this chapter. You want to tell the Deaf person that you are studying and learning to sign in ASL, that you are excited to work with them, and you hope the two of you will be friends. Go ahead; you know the signs. Follow the ASL gloss below. A *gloss* shows the order of the signs but represents neither an English sentence nor the complete syntax of ASL. Remember, ASL is not a written language and can only be appreciated fully in three dimensions. Glosses are a simple written tool for recording sign order. Try it out; add the appropriate facial expressions!

**ME   LEARN   ASL   EXCITED   YOU   WORK
TWO-OF-US   FRIENDS**

EXERCISES

Hearing people can learn to communicate with Deaf people by using their eyes, bodies, and hands when signing in ASL. Deaf people, however, cannot learn to communicate with hearing people by using their ears. Here are two exercises that will help you get in touch with the Deaf experience.

Sounds Like

Imagine you are standing under a beautiful waterfall with a Deaf friend. How would you show that sound to your friend? What facial expressions, body movements, and gestures would you use?

How can you show visually, something you hear? Try to show the following situations.

- The fuzzy snowlike background when a TV station's regularly scheduled programming has ended.
- The crack a bat makes when it hits a baseball.
- Classical music. Jazz. Rock music.
- Cars moving on the freeway.
- Laughter.

Shopping Trip

What must it be like to find basic communication with people in your community difficult? As a person sensitive to this concern, you may want to experience firsthand the kinds of challenges that sometimes arise for a Deaf person in hearing society. Go on a shopping trip. You might want to bring your signing partner along to help you with this exercise.

1. Choose a day when you would ordinarily go shopping.

2. Make a list of where you will be shopping and what you will need to buy.

3. Bring a friend, family member, or preferably, your sign partner with you.

4. Go to each store and purchase your items. Wear earplugs to muffle incoming sounds and do not talk out loud. Use any way you can to communicate—pointing, gesturing, and mouthing words. Avoid writing things down or letting your companion speak for you.

The same exercise can be done in a group at home or in a classroom setting by playing store: Set up an office supply store, bakery, and shoe store. Have group members gesturally describe the items they want to purchase. Divide the group into shoppers and store clerks, and enjoy your shopping spree!

Now, we are ready to make our way in the world, communicating in sign with a heightened awareness of the Deaf experience and Deaf culture. Let's take a closer look in the next chapter at how people come together and move apart. What are the proper customs and etiquette for meeting someone new? How do you join an ASL conversation? Interrupt a conversation? End a conversation and break eye contact without seeming rude? As you'll see, the rules for Deaf culture are different from those for hearing society. Again, the key is to use your eyes, bodies, and hands—not your ears!

Additional Vocabulary

BEAUTIFUL. Place the dominant hand in front of your face, fingers spread and palm facing you. Move the hand across your face in a circular motion, bringing the fingertips together to touch the thumb as you complete the circle.

BELIEVE. Using the pointer finger of your dominant hand, touch your forehead. Then, using closed "C"-hands, bring your dominant palm to rest in your upturned palm, thumbs closing like clasping hands. This sign actually means "married to your thoughts."

COOPERATE. Touch the thumb and forefinger of one hand together, leaving your other fingers extended. Make the same handshape on your other hand. Lock the thumb and index fingers of both hands like a chain linked together. Move the hands forward in a circular motion in front of your body, palms facing each other and perpendicular to the body.

ENCOURAGE. Using both five-hands, palms facing out, gently push forward as if urging someone to move ahead.

GALLAUDET. As Dr. Gallaudet wore tiny spectacles, his name sign became a description of his glasses and is used today to refer to Gallaudet University. Using the forefinger and thumb of your dominant hand, the other fingers remaining in a fist, bring your hand in front of your eye where glasses frames would be and touch the thumb and forefinger together.

IMAGINE. Place both hands in front of your forehead in the "C" or "claw" handshape, palms facing each other. Move the hands away from each other while opening your fingers. This is called the dream bubble. It can be used just before you explain a dream for your future goals or to pretend something.

INTRODUCE. Place both flat five-hands, fingers closed, about hip-width apart, elbows bent, and palms facing up toward the ceiling. Move the hands together in front of you to touch the tips of the middle fingers together.

OFFER. Open both hands, palms upturned, fingers together. Move both hands up and out as if you had a tray or a book you are offering to someone in front of you.

RESPECT. Cross the forefinger and third finger of both hands, as in keeping your fingers crossed. Bring the hands in front of your forehead and then out away from the body. This is a directional sign and should be aimed toward the person to whom respect is given.

RESPONSIBILITY. Bend the flat five-hands and touch the fingertips of both hands to the nondominant shoulder. Imagine you are placing a weight on your shoulders.

SHARE. Place both five-hands in front of the body, palms facing you with thumbs pointing up. Move your dominant hand so that the pinky finger side touches the forefinger side of the nondominant hand. Move the dominant hand back and forth across the topside of the non-dominant forefinger and between the upturned thumb.

SOUL. Touching the thumbs and forefingers together, leave the other fingers extended. Place your nondominant hand in front of your stomach, palm facing in. Take your dominant hand and move it, using the same handshape, in a fluttering motion as if ascending to the heavens.

SUCCESS. Using the pointer fingers of both hands, touch the corners of your mouth. Turn the hands, palms now facing out in front of you, to point both extended pointer fingers straight up into the air.

Chapter **5**

Meetings and Greetings

The first step to initiate a conversation in American Sign Language (ASL) is to establish eye contact with another person. You must be able to see one another to converse freely. This may seem easy, but think about it. A hearing person can call out from another room, turn away in the middle of a task, or convey a nuance of expression or emotion simply by modulating their tone of voice and still get the correct message across. Conversation in ASL, however, depends on the visual connection of two or more people.

Eye to Eye

Fluent ASL signers have trained themselves to focus their attention on the speaker while filtering in an awareness of the environment around them. Hearing people are not similarly trained to sustain eye contact while taking note of peripheral details. Dependent on the ear, hearing people are habituated to look around and constantly shift attention; they can pay attention with the ear as well as they can with the eye.

So, eye contact is not necessary for a hearing person to understand someone or even to convey that they are truly listening to the speaker. Moreover, staring is often considered rude in hearing society. The intensity of close observation is thought to be intrusive, an invasion of privacy.

For Deaf people, holding eye contact is the one basic essential to understanding; conversation cannot happen without it. Breaking eye contact signals an end to communication. The intensity of this position is clear in the formal signs for "look away" and "look at me."

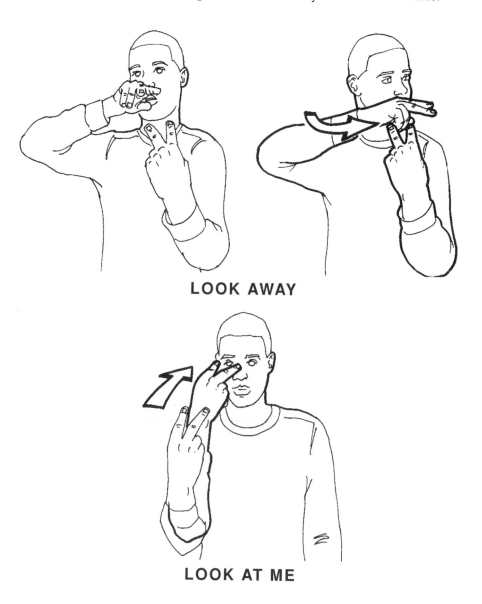

LOOK AWAY

LOOK AT ME

In the formal sign for "look away" we see the attention of the speaker initially oriented as a mirror image of the watching set of eyes represented by the "V" of the nondominant hand. Note that the hand-shape is the same for both hands. Then, the dominant hand changes location, movement, and palm orientation; the head turns to literally break eye contact, yet the nondominant hand remains stationary. The visual connection is severed; communication is not possible. Similarly, the formal sign for "look at me" is equally sharp. The location of the sign moves in the direction of the speaker and the focus centers on the eyes: "Pay attention. Look at me."

When conversing in ASL the focus between the participants remains steady on the face and eyes. As beginning signers, however, many people will tend to look more closely at someone's hands than their face. Remember the five basic components of ASL that we learned in Chapter 1 and their order of importance: (1) eye contact, (2) facial expression, (3) body language, (4) mouth movements, and (5) hand movements. Eye contact is the most important! With a partner, practice the art of visually perceiving signs. Try to order your visual perception to match the order of importance of the five basic components of ASL. If, for example, you only look at hand movements, you might miss a crucial facial expression that alters the meaning of the sign performed. Consider the sign for "meet" (on page 42). If you look too closely at the hands and miss your partner's head shaking no simultaneously, you will misunderstand them—your partner is actually communicating, "did not meet." So, the locus of attention when signing *always* begins on the face and eyes and moves outward to encompass the hands and upper body.

Take advantage of every opportunity to watch fluent signers converse in ASL. You'll learn a lot from studying how they use the five basic components of ASL to communicate efficiently and effectively, and you'll develop strong observation skills that will help you focus your attention properly when understanding ASL in conversation.

Excuse Me

How many times have you brushed up against someone inadvertently to get past them while walking down a hallway or corridor at

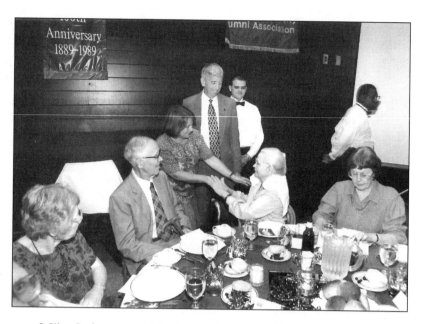

I. King Jordan (center) joins in conversation at the Gallaudet Alumni Association's 100th anniversary reception. Notice the strong eye contact as friends gather to share news of their daily lives.

school or at work and, in doing so, interrupted their conversation? Invariably, the person will turn in your direction as you brush by. "Excuse me," you say. Or what about walking between people as they are talking? Instinctively, you might tend to duck down as you pass and again say, "Excuse me." This is the proper etiquette of hearing society, as Dear Abby or Miss Manners will readily agree. But let's examine the motivation for this fundamental social custom. The cues for our response of "Excuse me" all depend on the sense of hearing! You *hear* someone coming up behind you; you are conditioned to *look* in the direction of the sound. You make yourself smaller as you pass between two conversing people to minimalize the visual distraction, but the speakers can still *hear* each other—you have not disrupted their ability to continue their conversation, and your softly spoken apology is merely an acknowledged piece of background noise.

Suppose you are interrupting a conversation in ASL? What then? When you sign "Excuse me" you will break the eye contact of the two Deaf signers. How can you pass through without disturbing them? The socially acceptable thing to do is to walk as unobtrusively between the signers as possible. Acknowledging your presence in their visual field by ducking down or by drawing the eye contact of one or both of the signers is distracting. A Deaf person will understand that most hearing people may not know the importance of eye contact for communication in ASL. We, however, can now avoid such a "hearing-minded" mistake.

Let's say your new Deaf coworker from Chapter 4 has invited you to come along to a party at a Deaf friend's house. You are making your way through the congenial gathering of hearing and Deaf partygoers. As you approach the hors d'oeuvres table, you realize that you must brush up against a Deaf person absorbed in a conversation. Okay, *now* what do you do? Surely, if you nudge the Deaf person lightly on the shoulder in the direction you wish them to move, you think you will disturb their conversation and receive a stern facial expression of disapproval. But don't worry—respectfully nudging the shoulder is the acceptable thing to do in this case. Deaf people use touch as an important way to give and receive cues for movement and to stay aware of what is happening around them. Unlike a hearing person, who will *turn* in the direction of the touch, a Deaf person will *move* in the direction of the touch. The signers will shift their position to let you pass without needing to glance in your direction.

Joining In

Now that you've enjoyed a tasty hors d'ouevre, you'd like to join in the signed conversation. You might want to tap one of the signers on the arm or gently tug their arm in your direction. Even simpler, wait for an appropriate moment and establish eye contact. If the signers are several feet away from you, you might want to engage their attention as you approach by extending one arm in front of you and waving your hand up and down.

In their first encounters with Deaf people, hearing people often make a few common mistakes. The most common involves exaggerated movements. Deaf people are connoisseurs of visual observation; actors could study the intricate and subtle facial expressions of a fluent ASL signer and admire a Deaf person's highly developed ability to process and evaluate what they see. Waving your hand in a Deaf person's face is considered an annoyance, as are overdone facial expressions and elaborate mouth movements intended to help the Deaf

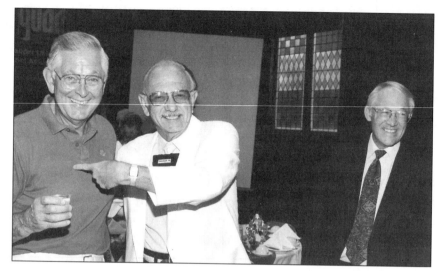

Three Deaf community leaders, Dr. Victor Galloway (left), Dr.Gerald "Bummy" Burstein (center), and Dr. Jack R. Gannon (right), share a laugh.

person lipread. All are unneccesary. The best way to approach conversing with a Deaf person is to have respect and consideration and to forget about your hearing-mind. Follow the Deaf person's lead for the correct behavior and allow them to guide you through the proper etiquette for conversation. You are a hearing person who has entered the environment of Deaf culture—you'll need to *look* and *feel* your way around. You'll find you are beginning to trust more than your sense of hearing to communicate and to process your thoughts and feelings.

There, you've established eye contact with the Deaf couple by the hors d'oeuvres table. They are gesturing for you to join in their conversation. But wait a minute. What about personal space? We know it is acceptable for people to touch each other in the Deaf community, but how close is too close? In general, you want to maintain a comfortable distance, usually about three feet, so that signers can move easily. Equally important, however, the space gives the Deaf person enough distance to properly view signs without the eye strain of standing up too close or back too far. Just as hearing people naturally adjust the loudness of their voices to suit different environments, Deaf people will adjust their stances appropriately to allow for the most effective communication under varying conditions. Signing often becomes quite a challenge when one of you is munching on chips and salsa and the other is drinking a glass of seltzer; you both have to sign with one hand. Spills are frequent and dismissed as a matter of course. There is a far greater tolerance in the Deaf community for a looser sense of touch and personal space. While you must have enough room to maintain proper eye contact, the experience of personal space is far less proprietary than is usually found among hearing people.

Introductions

As you join in conversation with your new Deaf friends, they ask you if you are hearing, where you learned to sign, and whether you have any Deaf family, friends, or coworkers. They may also ask you where you live, where you attend school, or where you work. There is one thing, however, they seem to leave out of their questions. Can you guess what it is? Of course, it is the first question a hearing person will ask another hearing person upon meeting them for the first time: "What is your name?"

In hearing society people are taught that finding out someone's name, memorizing it, and repeating it often in conversation are essential communication skills that build trust and intimacy. Most hearing people would find it odd and even rude for another person to begin talking without introducing themselves by name or without asking you for your name in return. But, once more, we must come back to the visual to understand the perspective of introductions in Deaf culture. Deaf people identify each other through *description*. The *picture* becomes the *name*. When a Deaf person meets someone new, observing their appearance and learning about their circumstances is the equivalent of "naming" them. A Deaf person will want to know first if you are hearing or Deaf. Then they will want to know where you, a hearing person, learned to sign and perhaps how many years you have been using ASL. This information is very important for communication purposes because it reveals how much experience you have signing in ASL. For a hearing person, several years of learning ASL in a program taught by Deaf instructors shows a respect for Deaf culture and indicates that you will use signs correctly—particularly if you studied at Gallaudet! Next, you will be asked whether your parents are Deaf and who your Deaf family, friends, or coworkers are. Establishing your connections to other Deaf people places you within the Deaf community and gives the Deaf person a context for your involvement in Deaf culture. Further, knowing where you live, attend school, or work places you *physically* within the Deaf community. This is another potential link that can connect you to common acquaintances with your new Deaf friend. For example, many Deaf people hold government jobs in the United States, because this country's government is very progressive about hiring Deaf workers. Perhaps you may know some of the same people. (In Japan, the opposite is true; there are more incentives in the private sector for Deaf workers.)

All of this information—whether you're hearing or Deaf, where you learned to sign, and if your parents or friends are Deaf—is immediately exchanged in the first moments of introduction. You see, your English name is really the least important thing that describes you. It is not a part of the *picture*. In the way that listening to the sound of their names is a pleasant experience that establishes a link between two hearing people, the visual contact, face to face, establishes the link between two Deaf people. Later, your new Deaf friends might meet your Deaf coworker and ask them about you: "How is that tall, brunette woman (man) with glasses who works with you and is learning to sign? You brought her (him) to the party?" "Yes . . ." Your English name may or may not be mentioned.

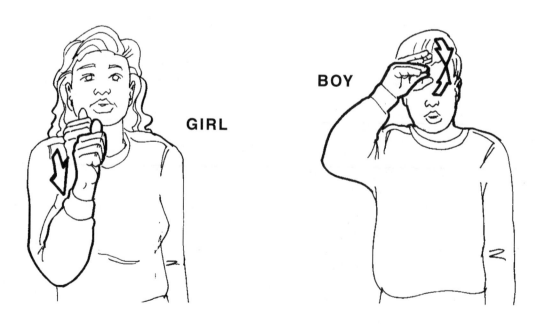

GIRL

BOY

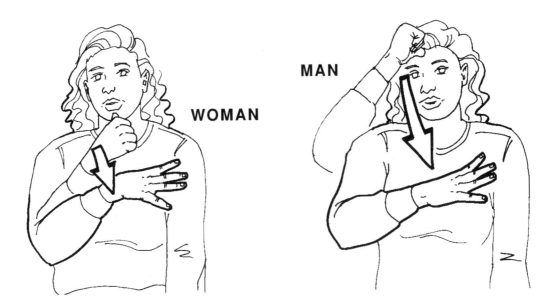

WOMAN

MAN

The signs for "girl," "boy," "woman," and "man" are important for describing someone to another person. They instantly convey age and gender. Go back to the "yellow room in the house" from Chapter 2; remember that we must see the house before we can see the room. The first picture communicated is the most basic identifying one for context. Establishing age and gender are the most basic descriptors we can use to see a person. Then, other physical and circumstantial characteristics—"tall," "brunette," "glasses," "coworker," "student of ASL," "met at the party"—will be used to fill in the details until recognition is achieved.

Do Deaf people ever use English names, you are wondering. They must have to use them to get around in hearing society. Absolutely. You are right. Deaf people do understand that names are important to hearing people. At the end of a conversation, you may want to exchange business cards with a Deaf person. If you have a sign language interpreter for your conversation, they will voice the Deaf person's name for you and fingerspell your name for the Deaf person. If you do not have a sign language interpreter, you will want to write your name down on a piece of paper for the Deaf person and ask them to do the same for you.

Usually, Deaf people use English names only in very formal conversational settings, or when a document such as a lease or contract needs their signature. The formal ASL sign for "name" refers to the written English name.

NAME. Using the middle and index fingers of both hands as extended pointer fingers, the index fingers facing the ceiling and the palms facing each other, stack the fingers of the dominant hand over the fingers of the nondominant hand to form an "X." The "X" represents the written signature of an English name.

TO SIGN (A DOCUMENT). Make a flat page with the nondominant five-hand, fingers together and palm facing up. The pointing index and middle fingers of the dominant hand, index finger facing toward the ceiling, come down to tap the extended fingers and then the open palm of the page hand: "Sign here."

Sometimes, Deaf people will give each other name signs that usually refer to some defining characteristic of a person. The author of this book, Diane Chambers, received her name sign from Deaf children at the Maryland School for the Deaf where she once worked. Because of her curly hair, the children gave her this name sign: With the dominant hand, make a fist and extend the pointer finger toward the ceiling; touch the tips of the three fist fingers to the thumb. This is the signed letter for "D." Place the hand up by the hair and circle it in a downward motion next to the hair and face to show brushing curls. See how the visual perception of the person identifies them in sign! The name sign is so highly personalized that you must know the person to understand the sign. Fingerspelling English names is awkward and impersonal in Deaf culture and is sometimes avoided. If someone does not know your name sign, it would still be preferable to describe you: "You know, the sign language interpreter with the curly hair? She interpreted for the business meeting last month? She wrote a book about ASL and Deaf culture. She lives in Baltimore." "Yes . . ."

A common name sign for many Deaf people is the signed letter for their first initial placed on the chest, where a name tag might appear. The editor of this book, Keith Robertson, received this name sign from his classmates at Deaf residential school. With the dominant hand, extend the index and middle fingers toward the ceiling and place the thumb between them, also facing toward the ceiling. The other two fingers bend down toward the palm. This is the signed letter "K." Place the "K" on the chest with palm facing in.

Remember, a name sign can only be given to you by a Deaf person.

How are you?

"How is that tall, brunette woman (man) with glasses who works with you and is learning to sign? You brought her (him) to the party?" "Yes . . ."
This is the way a sign language interpreter might voice in English the question your new Deaf friends from the party are asking your Deaf coworker. It follows the linear rules of a good English sentence. But as we are learning, the three dimensions of ASL require a different syntax, grammar, and sign order. It is possible to sign "How are you?" in English word order. In fact, a Deaf person can easily spot a hearing person by their insistence on signing this sentence in English word order. Deaf people tend not to use this construction. Its intangible quality does not translate well into the picture language of ASL. A closer English translation of what Deaf people will sign to each other is "How do you feel?"

FEEL. Use your dominant five-hand with fingers spread apart and extended. Bend the middle finger in slightly, with the palm facing your chest. Touch the middle finger lightly to your heart and rub the finger over it. The basic handshape for "feel" resonates with meaning in ASL; it is a common element of many formal ASL signs concerning feelings and emotions.

HOW DO YOU FEEL? Using the handshape for "feel," take both hands and touch the middle fingers lightly to the chest. Brush the middle fingers up off the chest and out in front of your body. This sign can also be used to mean "What's up?," "What's happening?," or "What's new?"; or it can refer to a specific event—as in "I went to the 'event'; it was a party." The specific meaning of the sign, then, will come from its context in conversation.

The English sentence *How are you?* does not work in ASL because the verb *to be* is used in a different way in sign language. As a linear language, *to be* takes on a vital purpose in building sentences in English.

Because of its visual and spatial orientation, however, ASL does not need to rely on "to be" to link noun subjects to verbs, and the construction has a very limited function in sign language. *Am, is, was,* and *are* are all formed in a different way in ASL. The formal sign for "are" takes on a very literal meaning of "real," as in "it is being" or "it exists." The sign describes the state of being, much as Hamlet meant it in his famous soliloquy on existence that begins "To be or not to be: that is the question."

REAL. The extended pointer finger of the dominant hand touches the mouth and moves forward away from the face.

To be, as a linking verb, then, is unnecessary in ASL. It has no *picture.* If someone wanted to ask you, "Are you tired?" they would sign

TIRED   YOU

and add a questioning facial expression. The linking verb is already contained in the signed question, to sign it formally would be clumsy and inefficient. You can even convey the question by signing just "tired" with the proper facial expression. Here, the signer's facial expression functions as tone of voice and inflection would for the same abbreviated question voiced in English.

Because Deaf people do not use *to be* in ASL, their written English may not make use of this linking verb as well. The Deaf person may still have a strong command of the English language and the mistake should not be interpreted by hearing people as an inability to understand and use English—it is just that the way verbs are constructed is totally different in ASL than it is in English. When a hearing person signs "How are you?" in English word order to a Deaf person, they are really making an equivalent grammatical error in ASL! ASL and English are two distinct languages with different rules for building sentences.

The answer to the question, "How do you feel?" is "Fine."

FINE. The dominant five-hand with fingers extended points out away from the body with the thumb facing up toward the ceiling. Bring the thumb toward the body to touch the breast bone. If you are feeling great, brush the hand up and out again, thumb once more toward the ceiling, for an emphatic response.

Saying Good-Bye

The party is winding to a close and your Deaf friend gestures that it is time to say good-bye. You have made many new friends at the party, Deaf and hearing, particularly the Deaf couple by the hors d'ouevres table who, you've discovered, both work for a different division of your parent company. Their Deaf son goes to the same school your Deaf coworker attended growing up. Their hearing daughter takes in-line skating classes at a park near your home. You nod to your friend to acknowledge that it is time to go, and begin the process of saying good-bye to all of your new friends. As you move from conversation to conversation, you make a "thumb's up" sign before breaking eye contact and approaching the next person. You are careful to hold eye contact until you know the Deaf person has acknowledged the mutual end of your conversation and you know it is okay to look away. If you remember something you need to ask someone, "What time are we going to meet to watch the football game on TV next Monday night?," just tap the person on the shoulder to reestablish eye contact. If the person has already moved across the room, no problem . . . wave! This is perfectly acceptable in Deaf culture. Unlike hearing society, Deaf people can converse easily across the distance of a room as long as sight lines are clear. The only issue becomes privacy—everyone can see what you are signing. For a private conversation, move where other people cannot see you. Sometimes even this is not enough to ensure privacy. Suppose you are walking down the hallway to get your coat and discover two people who have moved there to have a private conversation. Just walk quickly by without establishing eye contact or acknowledging the signers. You can usually tell when two people want privacy by watching their body language. If they are walking in front of you and slow down or shift their bodies away from you, take the hint and move on.

In the past, good-byes in Deaf culture often took as long as an hour. Before technology such as TTYs made communication from the home easier, social gatherings functioned as an important forum for exchanging information with others. People needed to convey as much as they could because they sometimes did not know how soon they would see each other again to converse face to face in ASL. One sign language interpreter, the daughter of Deaf parents, recalls more than once falling asleep in her coat with her brother and sister while waiting for her parents to say good-bye to friends at the end of a party. Use the opportunity, a long good-bye lets your Deaf friends know you support the Deaf community, enjoy their company, and look forward to seeing them again. Hugs and kisses are the norm. You will miss their companionship!

NICE TO MEET YOU. Perform the sign for "meet" (on page 42), but orient the sign so that the backs of the hands are facing the two signers. You are drawing the face-to-face connection between two people.

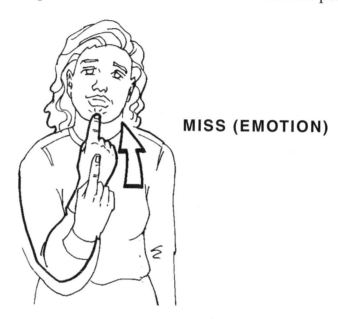

MISS (EMOTION)

EXERCISES

These exercises are fun ones. They will help you understand the way Deaf people rely on touch in social or group settings and to practice the art of naming friends, family, and coworkers by describing them visually.

Silent Dance

This exercise focuses on touch and motion during ASL conversations. Until you've actually experienced the physical rhythm, movement, and focus of eye contact while signing in ASL from the perspective of a Deaf person, you will always fall back subconsciously on your instinctive use of the hearing sense. Walking through a crowded room of Deaf people is much like the scene in the movie *The Fisher King*, where Robin Williams follows Amanda Plummer through a sea of moving bodies in New York's Grand Central Station and the movement takes on the qualities of a silent dance. In fact, the best way to experience this exercise is to put yourself in an all-Deaf environment. You'll quickly lose the need to listen with your ears or speak with your vocal chords as you *feel* your way around the room.

1. Take the last fifteen or twenty minutes of your sign study group to have an informal social get-together. If possible, move your group out of the classroom and into a more relaxed place, such as a student lounge, living room, outdoor setting, or restaurant.
2. Everyone must use ASL exclusively. No English allowed.
3. Everyone wears earplugs to muffle outside noise as much as possible.
4. Party on, using the etiquette of Deaf culture to guide your conversations. Notice how light or heavy your touch needs to be to move someone gently, to direct their attention, or to get it. Concentrate on ways of establishing and breaking eye contact between signers.
5. Ask a Deaf friend or two to attend your get-together as observers. At the end of the party, have the Deaf person(s) give pointers and advice or maybe even demonstrate some common techniques for using touch and movement to stay aware of the surrounding environment.

A Rose by Any Other Name

Practice the art of describing someone visually with natural gestures or formal ASL signs without using their English name. Use the formal signs listed in the "Additional Vocabulary" (on page 78) to help with this exercise.

1. In a group, gather into a circle. One person begins by describing the person to their right for the rest of the group. Use as

many natural gestures and formal ASL signs as you can to create a full detailed picture.

2. Continue around the circle with each group member describing the person to their right until everyone has been described.

Challenge 1: Now, continue around the circle again. This time each person chooses another group member at random to describe. The other members must identify who it is.

Challenge 2: Place two group members whose physical characteristics are similar in the center of the circle. How would you describe them so that others would recognize the right person?

Continue the exercise at home by describing family members with natural gestures and formal ASL signs to your spouse, partner, or parents. See how many they can identify!

In this chapter we've learned much about what it is like to converse with someone in ASL and have worked hard to increase our awareness of the Deaf experience. In the next chapter, let's visit a Deaf family at home. What time did our Deaf friends say that football game started?

Additional Vocabulary

AFRICAN AMERICAN. Make the sign for "Africa." Take the dominant hand and extend it in the five-hand handshape, palm facing out. Move the hand in a clockwise arcing motion bringing the fingers together at the bottom of the arc. You are drawing the map of Africa.

In the past, signs for ethnic and racial groups depicted the visual characteristics of that group. The traditional sign for African American was the sign for, literally, "black person." Our nation's growing multicultural sensitivity has led to a reevaluation of these signs, many of which are now based on maps, as in the sign for African American given above.

The sign for Caucasian remains centered on the visual. Perform the sign for the color "white": With the dominant five-hand, all fingers touch the chest and pull upward toward the throat as you close them together. The sign comes from the image of buttoning a white shirt. The sign for "white person" uses both hands and continues the motion to open the fingers onto the face, palms oriented inward.

BEARD. With the dominant hand, pull down from the chin to draw a goatee.

BROAD/MUSCULAR. With elbows bent at your sides, extend your forearms with hands in fists, thumb oriented toward the ceiling. With the thumb and forefinger of each hand, make an open C-shape. Move the hands up and out by the shoulders, elbows still bent, while puffing out your cheeks. Picture a large-chested Arnold or Sly!

CURLY HAIR. Use the dominant five-hand with fingers spread in a claw position and circle around your hair.

EYEGLASSES. With both hands, make the open C-shape with the index finger and thumb, the other fingers are bent toward the palm. Hold the open "C"-hands up to frame your eyes like a pair of glasses.

HAIR COLOR.

BLACK. The extended pointer finger of the dominant hand moves across the eyebrows, left to right if right-handed, and right to left if left-handed. The sign uses dark eyebrows to show "black." Catch a strand of hair between your thumb and index finger in the "okay" handshape for "black hair."

BLOND. Make the signed letter "Y" by extending the thumb and pinky finger of the dominant hand and touching the other fingers to the palm. Take the "Y"-hand beside the face, palm facing the cheek, and pull it down beside the hair without touching, rotating the hand slightly from the wrist to shake the "Y" as you move. This is literally "yellow hair."

BRUNETTE. Make the signed letter for "B" by taking the dominant flat five-hand and pulling the thumb across the palm. Move the "B"-hand down the side of the cheek, touching slightly. This is the sign for "brown" and originates as a reference to skin color. Then, make the "okay" handshape, catching a strand of hair between your thumb and forefinger for "brown hair."

GRAY. With both hands in front of you, take the five-hands with fingers spread and thumbs facing up, palms toward the body, and intertwine the fingers repeatedly. Literally, the sign shows mixing colors or muddying them. Catch a strand of hair between the thumb and index finger in the "okay" handshape to show "gray hair."

REDHEAD. The dominant forefinger touches the chin to scratch it just below the lips for "red." This comes from red lips. Catch a strand of hair between the thumb and forefinger with the "okay" handshape to show "red hair" or "redhead."

MUSTACHE. Place the index finger of your dominant hand over your upper lip.

OLD. Place the dominant fist under the chin, thumb touches chin, and pull it down to the stomach to draw a long, long beard in the air.

ROSY CHEEKED. Perform the sign for "red" (see above) and then touch the cheeks.

TALL. Place the nondominant five-hand in front of the body, fingers together, palm facing out away from you. The extended pointer finger of the dominant hand brushes against the palm in an upward motion.

THIN. Pinky fingers touch at the tip and draw a vertical line in the air, dominant hand on top. Suck in your breath and purse your lips.

YOUNG. With both hands, take the five-hand with fingers together and touch the fingertips to the chest high up near the shoulder. Brush the fingers upward in a repeated motion.

6

At Home

What better place than home to see how American Sign Language (ASL) is used every day. For many years, before ASL was recognized as a language in its own right, Deaf people described using sign language as "the way we communicate at home." Removed from the society at large—remember ASL was excluded from the educational environment after the 1880 Milan Conference—sign language evolved and flourished in the homes of Deaf families and the dormitories of residential schools for the Deaf. Today, Deaf families are proud to share their language and culture, deeply rooted in a strong home and community identity, with hearing society. The vibrancy, expressiveness, and emotion evident in ASL can be traced back to the everyday communications between loved ones in a Deaf family at home.

Introducing the Family

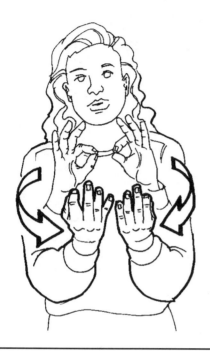

FAMILY. The Deaf community cherishes close-knit face-to-face interactions. The formal sign for "family" is based on the sign for group—a circle where the palms are oriented toward one another, as if to draw the family close around you.

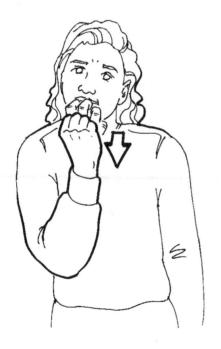

CARE. The facial expression for "care" is one of tenderness and compassion.

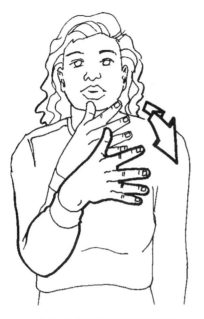

GRANDMOTHER

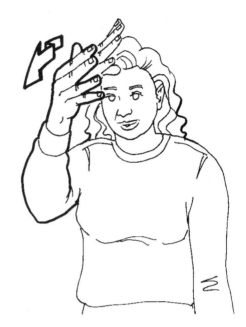

GRANDFATHER

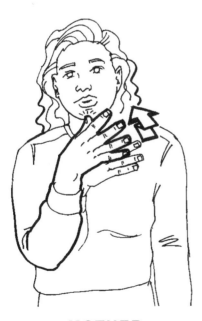

MOTHER

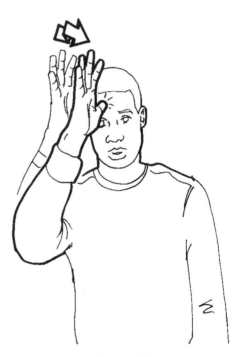

FATHER

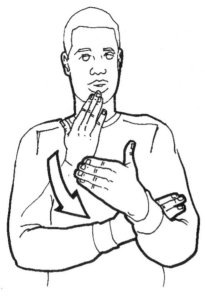

DAUGHTER

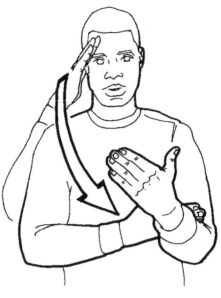

SON

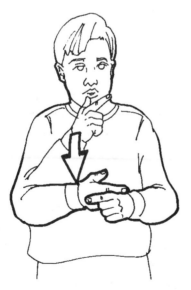

SISTER

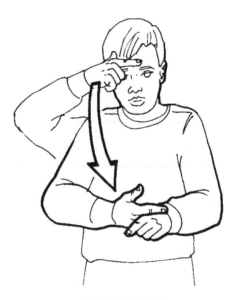

BROTHER

The formal signs for "mother" and "grandmother" use the same handshape, except that the movement for "mother" brings the thumb *toward* the chin while the movement for "grandmother" moves the thumb *away* from the chin, bouncing the hand once in the air to show the concept of a generation removed from the signer. The same thing happens with the signs for "father" and "grandfather."

The signs for "daughter," "son," "sister," and "brother," find their origin in performing the signs for "girl" and "boy" (on page 70) and then the sign for "baby." Over the years, "girl baby" and "boy baby" evolved to form the more efficient formal signs you see illustrated. Note that masculine signs generally begin at the forehead and feminine ones at the chin.

BABY. With flat five-hands, palms facing up, lay the back of the dominant hand on the base arm and rock the arms back and forth as if cradling an infant.

Make Yourself at Home

In the intimate environment of the home, a Deaf family must use ASL and rely on visual and tactile cues to converse with one another and go about the daily activities of living. As in all other aspects of the Deaf experience, seeing and feeling are the primary senses of understanding. Let's go visit a Deaf family to see and feel for ourselves.

As you arrive at your new Deaf friend's house, you know you are ready for a fun adventure. You begin to picture how the home ground can be a challenging environment where Deaf people must accommodate for many of the experiences of daily living that hearing people take for granted. How many features of the home are geared for hearing consumers? How do deaf people watch TV? Have telephone conversations? Answer the doorbell?

With your mind's eye, take a walk through your own house or apartment and identify activities that depend on the hearing sense. Make a list of each one you can think of. Ask yourself: Which appliances or structures must be modified for comfort and ease in a world of silence? What might you want to do to make a Deaf person feel at home in your house?

As you are welcomed into the Deaf home, prepare yourself with an open-mindedness and flexibility that will allow you to learn a new way of doing things. In many cases, you may find the Deaf solution to be more practical and efficient than the way things are done in a hearing home. As ever, leave your hearing-mind at the door. Go ahead; push the doorbell. See what happens.

Opening the Door

How does the family know I am here? you wonder. How does this doorbell work? Your Deaf friends' daughter, a hearing high school student, answers the door. But you didn't hear any bell ring when you pushed the doorbell. She presses the doorbell again and points to a lamp in the living room that is flashing on and off. It is hooked up to a device that flashes the light when someone presses the doorbell. An additional device is often also placed upstairs in a hallway, bedroom, or other easily visible spot. It makes perfect sense; the visual cue signals a visitor's arrival.

By now, the whole family and all of their guests are assembled in the living room to greet you. You say hello to your hosts, the Deaf couple you met at the party in Chapter 5, and to your Deaf coworker who has also been invited to watch the football game. Several other Deaf people whom you have not met before are also here. You shake hands with each one, and everyone exchanges stories about how they know the Deaf couple and add a little bit about themselves. You are introduced to the couple's young son, who attends the day-program of a Deaf residential grade school in your area.

Dialogue

ASL Gloss

NICE TO MEET   FAMILY   FRIENDS   HOUSE
BEAUTIFUL   YOU   PROUD   ROOMS   SEE   ?

Note: Remember, an ASL gloss is only an artificial written representation of a three-dimensional language. When signing the dialogue in ASL, remember to use all five of its basic components: (1) eye contact, (2) facial expression, (3) body language, (4) mouth movements, and (5) hand movements.

English Translation

It is so nice to meet your family and friends. Your house is beautiful. You must be very proud of it. I'd love to have a tour.

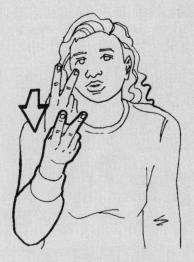

SEE/LET ME SEE

As your hosts show you from room to room in the house you are eagerly on the lookout for clues that reveal how the environment matches the needs to the Deaf family. The first thing you see is that the entire first floor of the house is very open and airy. The kitchen has a cut-out space in the wall with shutters that open and close onto the dining room; it also has a separate entrance to the living room. The dining room opens onto the living room, too. Of course, you realize, in a Deaf home communication is made easier by opening up common spaces and allowing people to see each other as they move from room to room. By waving or flicking a light switch, you can easily get some-one's attention.

As you climb the stairs to the second floor, you are reminded why some Deaf people often laugh during horror movies. Suddenly, it makes sense. If you turn the sound off during a horror movie and simply watch scenes of someone climbing to the landing and walking a hallway to open a bedroom door—well, what's so scary about that? When a monster appears, it seems silly. The suspense is signaled to hearing people through the frightening music that accompanies the scenes.

At the top of the stairs each door is opened to reveal the bedrooms—no ghosts playing hide and seek inside—and you ask your hostess what kind of alarm clock they use to get up in time for work each morning. There are two kinds. One makes use of a light that grows brighter and brighter to mimic the rising of the sun until it awakens you. The other is a vibrating alarm placed under the pillow or mattress that shakes you awake. Of course, there is always the gentle tap on the shoulder from someone who is already up and ready to start the day. Deaf people are more sensitive to touch than hearing people; touch alarms will easily awaken them.

"How does a Deaf mother know when her toddler or infant is crying?" you ask. Cry alarms, based on the sounds the baby or child makes, are hooked up to the living room and bedroom lights. When the child cries, the light flashes. "How can you distinguish a cry alarm flash from the doorbell?" Either the alarm is hooked up to a different light in each room or the flash is timed so that it looks different—much the same way alarms for hearing people *sound* different. Before technology made cry alarms possible, mothers used creative ways to keep an eye on their children. Some tied strings around the child's toe and their own wrist or ankle. When the baby cried and kicked, the mother felt it. Sometimes mothers put the baby's crib next to the parents' bed and slept with a hand in the crib.

Here are the formal signs for the rooms we have visited. For each sign, follow the description below and then perform the formal sign for "room," which you have already learned (on page 30).

LIVING ROOM. You will make the signs for "formal-room." The dominant five-hand, fingers spread apart, moves toward the body to bring the thumb to touch the chest. The thumb brushes upward and outward in a repeated circular motion to suggest the ruffles on a fancy shirt: formal. We are in a formal room or living room.

FAMILY ROOM. Perform the signs for "family-room" (see "family" on page 82).

KITCHEN. Make the signs for "cooking-room." Use the nondominant five-hand, palm up and fingers pointing out away from the body, as a base. Lay the dominant hand on top, palm facing down so the two palms touch each other, then flip the hand so the back of the palm touches. The motion resembles flipping pancakes, or turning food in a frying pan. This is the formal sign for "cook."

DINING ROOM. Perform the signs for "eat/food" and "room." Touch the thumb and fingers of the dominant hand together and bring them up to the mouth. This is the formal sign for "eat/food" (on page 93). The dining room is, literally, the "eating room."

BEDROOM. You will make the signs for "bed" and "room." Take the dominant flat five-hand and press the palm against the cheek, tilting the head toward the shoulder as the hand touches it. This is the formal sign for "bed."

What happens if no one in the family can see the doorbell flash to know that a visitor has arrived at their house? Patience and persistence are the concepts to remember. The visitor should look for a light on somewhere in the house. If a window to the lighted room is accessible, go to it and wave to get someone's attention. Check the yard. It if is dark, get a flashlight and flash it through the window. In a pinch, aim your headlights toward the house and flash them repeatedly. A common joke told in the Deaf community makes a clever—and humorous—turnaround of this technique for use in hearing society: A husband and wife check into a motel for the evening. Both are Deaf. The husband goes out to do some errands and returns only to find he does not remember which room is theirs. He honks the car horn until every light in the motel comes on except for one—his wife's. That's their room!

Using Telecommunications Devices for the Deaf and Telephone Relay Services

"How do I call without a TTY?" you ask.

Communication in the Deaf community is greatly facilitated by advances in technology that have made phone and written messages easy to send and receive via relay, TTY, fax, or beeper. Like alarm clocks, beepers are vibration activated. Today, you will often see pay phones in hotels, roadway rest stops, and airports equipped with TTY access. As a hearing person, however, you don't have to find a TTY to place a call to a Deaf person. Under the federal Americans with Disabilities Act, each state has been mandated to set up an operator relay system that you can use by calling an 800 number available by dialing Information. The operator will connect you with the TTY number you are calling and voice the TTY message of the Deaf person for you. When using relay services, remember to address the Deaf person directly—not the operator who is merely relaying the conversation. And be patient, there will be gaps and pauses while the operator relays to each party. A Deaf person can also use their TTY to call a hearing person through relay services.

TTYs (frequently referred to as TDDs in the hearing community) are devices that hook up to a standard telephone. Based on the old teletype machines, TTYs translate the telephone conversation into a typed message that appears on a screen. Some TTYs can print out the conversation as well. (Make sure a Deaf person knows that you are printing out a conversation and get their permission to do so.) A Deaf person recognizes that they have a phone call coming in because (like the doorbell) a light, often located in the kitchen or bedroom, will flash to let them know.

To place a TTY call, dial the number on the phone and place the receiver onto the TTY coupler—much like a computer modem. Some TTYs connect directly into the telephone hookup and do not require a coupler. When the other party answers, you will need to identify yourself immediately, HELLO DIANE HERE GA. GA means "go ahead." After the other party identifies who has answered the phone, you may begin conversing. Because two people cannot talk at the same time, you always want to give the other person the opportunity to make sure they have said everything they want to say before continuing. After every statement you make, type in GA. When you are ready to hang up, you will want to say that you need to go now and then you will type GA OR SK. When you type GA OR SK you are telling the other party that you are ready to hang up (stop keying) but are giving them a chance to add to the conversation if they desire to. As you might be able to guess, TTY conversations often continue well past the first GA OR SK as the callers move from one subject to another. Typing in SKSK means you are going to hang up. The other person will acknowledge by also typing SKSK. Don't hang up until the other person has confirmed the end of the conversation—they might have even more to say.

keith here ga

HI KEITH DIANE HERE GA   I AM CALLING U BACK GA

yes i called u about dinner tmw   can you come to the bbq q ga

YES   WHAT TIME Q GA

we will start cooking on grill at 4   probably ready to eat at 5 ga

OK I WILL SHOW UP AT 4:30 OK Q GA

fine ga

**I HAVE SOMETHING IMPT TO TELL U WHEN I SEE YOU
PREFER ASL GA**

**ok i need to go now i teach tonight ok see u tmw take care ga
or sk**

**OK SEE U TMW I LOOK FORWARD TO BBQ TAKE CARE GA OR
SK**

sure bye sksk

SKSK

TTY users make use of many abbreviations to speed up conversation. You may even type in HA HA or SMILE to show your emotion. It is impolite to read TTY conversations over someone's shoulder unless you are given permission. The caller would type MY FRIEND LEE ANN HAS NEVER SEEN A TTY CONVERSATION OK TO SHOW HER NOW Q GA. Of course, it is perfectly acceptable to tell other people in the room who it is you are conversing with on the TTY: "Lee Ann, Keith is on the phone."

Common TTY Abbreviations

ABT	about
AM/PM	morning/evening
CUL	see you later
CUZ	because
GA	go ahead
HAND	have a nice day
HD	hold
ILY	I love you
OIC	oh I see
PLS	please
Q	question
R	are
SK	stop keying
TMW	tomorrow
U	you
UR	your

Your friend's son is flicking the hall light to get your attention. Time to come downstairs and watch the football game.

Relaxing Together

The football game is about to begin. It is closed-captioned to show the commentary of the game announcers on the TV screen, much like the subtitles in a foreign-language film. The hosts and their guests settle in to enjoy a fun evening together. In the Deaf community, people gather regularly to watch events together on TV and to communicate face to face in ASL. When calling a Deaf person on the TTY during evening hours, remember that they may be using this opportunity to view a closed-captioned movie or program. Be considerate.

Dialogue

ASL Gloss

EAT   DRINK   WANT   ?   POPCORN   MICROWAVE   ?

Note: Remember, an ASL gloss is only an artificial written representation of a three-dimensional language. When signing the dialogue in ASL, remember to use all five of its basic components: (1) eye contact, (2) facial expression, (3) body language, (4) mouth movements, and (5) hand movements.

English Translation

Does anyone want something to eat or drink? Should we microwave some popcorn?

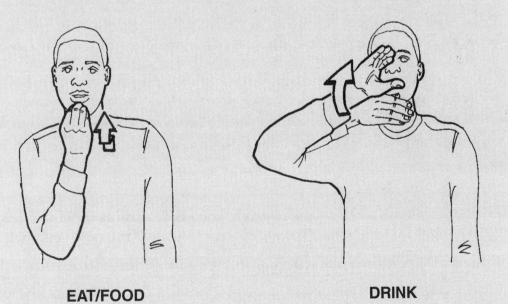

EAT/FOOD   DRINK

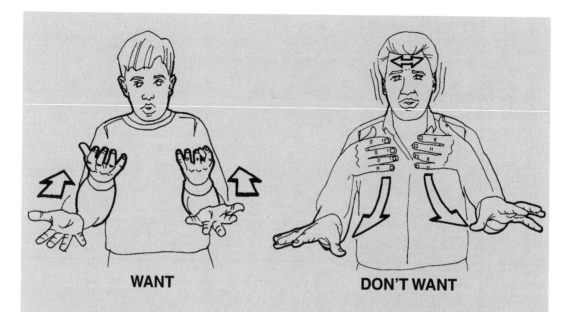

WANT **DON'T WANT**

POPCORN. Make fists with both hands and place them in front of you, palms facing toward the ceiling. Touch the index fingers to the thumbs. Flick one index finger upward while moving the whole hand up as well. Repeat with the other hand in an alternating fashion to show popcorn popping!

MICROWAVE. Touch the fingertips of both hands to the thumbs and hold the hands in front of the body with palms facing each other. Move the hands together while spreading the fingers into the open five-hand. As you move the hands, insert the fingers into the open spaces of the other hand. You are zapping food in the microwave. Repeat the motion.

As you snack on the popcorn, you ask your hosts about the formal signs for meal times. You are curious to know if the signs combine the concepts of "food" and "time of day" in the same way the formal signs for the rooms in the house combine "function" and "room." Yes, precisely! Meal times are signed by performing the formal sign for "eat," followed by the time of day: Sign "eat-morning" for "breakfast," "eat-noon" for "lunch," and "eat-night" for "dinner."

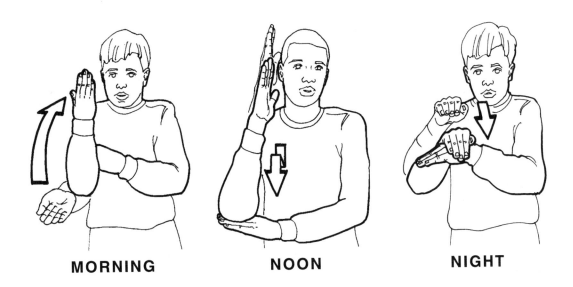

MORNING **NOON** **NIGHT**

You wait until your host looks up from the popcorn bowl to ask, continuing your line of reasoning, whether "snack" is signed by performing "eat-afternoon." No, your host informs you with a gentle smile, you'd just sign "eat-food" for "snack." But here's the formal sign for "afternoon."

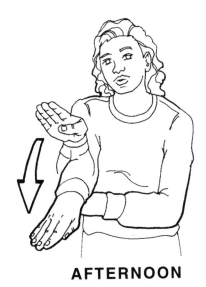

AFTERNOON

You've enjoyed your visit to your Deaf friends' home and look forward to returning soon. Already, you've begun to think about how you could make changes in your own home that would help your Deaf friends feel more comfortable when they come for a visit to *your* house! In the next chapter, we'll go on the job to explore the special needs of the workplace.

EXERCISES

Let's see how well you know your way around the house!

What Are You Doing?

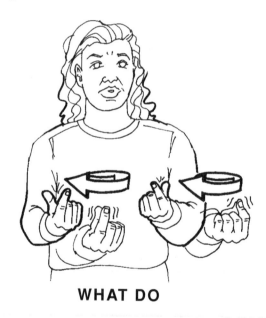

WHAT DO

This one formal sign actually depicts an entire concept: "What do you want to do?" or "What can I do?" (Usually this usage indicates a difficult situation, such as, "My friend isn't home to receive the package, what can I do?")

What do you do around the house? Go through each room of your house and think about what your daily routine is like. How would you describe this to a Deaf person? Describe furniture. Explain the function of appliances. Tell who lives at your house. Use formal signs and natural gestures, whatever you need to discuss with the Deaf person what your home is like and what you do there every day—from brushing your teeth in the morning to taking out the garbage after dinner. This exercise will help you to gain experience expressing common situations using basic elements of ASL.

Signing at Home

Practice translating the following English sentences into sign language. As always, make use of each component of ASL: (1) eye contact, (2) facial expression, (3) body language, (4) mouth movements, and (5) hand movements. Remember that the sign order will not be the same as the English word order. Which concepts need to be conveyed first?

1. Mom, I feel sick to my stomach from eating too much popcorn. I want to go to bed.
2. My brother and father are watching the football game. Do you want to go to the kitchen with me? My sister is cooking dinner.
3. My bedroom is yellow. I think it is beautiful. It is where I sleep and study.
4. Our white cat likes to drink milk and follow me to school.
5. My grandfather is old. He is proud of his gray hair. He enjoys going to movies with my grandmother.
6. We are happy to see our Deaf friends and practice signing.
7. I am thirsty. Let's drink a cup of tea in the family room.
8. The telephone is in my daughter's bedroom.
9. Imagine how hungry I am. I want to eat a big salad for lunch.
10. The teacher knows we are working hard to understand. She encourages us. We respect her.

Additional Vocabulary

CAKE. Place the nondominant hand as a base with the flat five-hand palm facing up. With the dominant hand in the "C" or "claw" handshape, touch the fingertips to the palm of the base hand and rotate the hand in a circular motion to show the round shape of a cake.

CHAIR/SIT. Make a fist with the nondominant hand and place it in front of your body, palm facing the floor. Extend the pointer and middle fingers. Using the same handshape, "sit" the pointer and middle fingers of the dominant hand on top of the base hand at a perpendicular angle. You may also curl the fingers over the side, as if the fingers are "sitting." Perform the motion one definitive time for "sit"; tap the fingers twice to show "chair."

DOCTOR/NURSE. Extend the nondominant hand as a base in the flat five-hand handshape, palm facing up and fingertips pointed outward. Touch the index and middle fingers of the dominant hand to the wrist of the base hand as if taking a pulse. This is the formal sign for "nurse." For "doctor," tap three fingers to the wrist.

DOOR. Place both flat five-hands in front of your body, thumbs touching and palms oriented outward. Rotate the dominant hand back and forth from the wrist to show a door opening and closing. To sign "open the door," swing the dominant hand to face the palm in toward the body. To sign "close the door," swing the dominant hand back in to touch the thumbs of both hands together again.

FOOTBALL. Hold both flat five-hands in front of the body, palms facing each other and thumbs toward the ceiling. Bring the hands together to lace the extended fingers. You are showing the players rushing into a scrimmage.

HOME. Perform the formal sign for "eat/food" (on page 93), but place it closer to the cheek than the mouth. Then, move the fingertips to touch the upper cheek. Home is, after all, where we eat and sleep, and this is where the sign originated.

HUSBAND. Hold the dominant hand in the "C" or "claw" handshape at the forehead, palm facing out. Move it downward to clasp the base hand at about chest height.

LAMP. With the dominant hand at eye level, touch fingertips to thumb. Move the fingers downward as they open out to show light shining from the lamp (see "sun" on page 30).

PETS. Sometimes pets are given English names, but oftentimes a Deaf person will describe their pet. They may refer to the pet using the sign for that animal.

BIRD. With the dominant hand, extend the thumb and index finger while touching the other fingers to the palm. Touch the back of the hand to the corner of the mouth. Bring the thumb and index finger to the corner of the mouth and close them together to form a beak.

If you are having chicken for dinner, you would make the sign for "bird."

CAT. Touch the thumb and forefinger of the dominant hand together, leaving the remaining fingers extended, and brush them out from the cheek. Repeat. You've grown whiskers!

DOG. Snap the fingers of the dominant hand and slap the thigh, as if calling your dog.

SALAD. With both hands in the "C" or "claw" handshape, fingers spread and palm facing up, move the hands as if tossing a salad.

SCHOOL. Place the nondominant flat five-hand in front of you, palm facing up and fingers pointing outward. Clap the other hand to cross it perpendicularly. How many times have you seen a teacher make this universal gesture to get students' attention?

SODA. With the nondominant hand, use the "C" or "claw" handshape to form the picture of a cup. With the dominant hand in a fist, extend the index finger and crook it. Pretend to flip back the top from an aluminum can of soda.

TEA. With the nondominant hand, use the "C" or "claw" handshape to form the picture of a cup. Touch the thumb and forefingers of the dominant hand together and dip the fingers repeatedly into the cup to show dipping a teabag.

TELEPHONE. The thumb and pinky finger of the dominant hand are extended, the other fingers touch the palm. Hold the thumb to the ear and finger to the mouth as if holding a receiver.

TTY (MAKE A CALL). With the nondominant hand, make a fist and extend the index finger to point straight out away from the body. Crook the index finger of the dominant hand and brush your nail along the other finger from knuckle to fingertip. This means "I'll call you on the TTY." The sign is directional; if you want someone to call you, reverse the movement in from the fingertip to the knuckle: "Call me on the TTY."

TV. Make a fist with the dominant hand and slip the thumb between the index and middle fingers. Hold the hand up with the palm facing away from the body. This is the signed letter for "T." Then extend the index and middle fingers toward the ceiling to form a "V," the signed letter for "V."

WATCH. Reverse the palm orientation of the handshape for "see" (on page 87) so that the palm faces away from the body and downward. Now the "V" of the eyes moves outward away from the body to show that you are watching something.

WIFE. Make the "C" or "claw" hand with both hands. With the dominant hand, palm facing down, touch the back of the hand to your chin. Move the hand down to clasp the upturned "C" of the nondominant hand.

Chapter 7

On the Job and at School

The connection between Deaf and hearing experiences is often made on the job or at school—two typical places in the community where Deaf and hearing people interact on a regular basis. The workplace and the classroom are excellent environments for hearing people to make Deaf friends and to learn more about sign language. The special demands of the office or classroom, where assignments and projects must be understood and completed, make it essential that good communication is established between everyone involved, whether Deaf or hearing! It is important for administrators and workers, teachers, parents, and students, to work together in a proactive collaboration to create an environment that is accessible for a Deaf person—one that stimulates their creativity and allows them to make a full contribution along with their hearing coworkers and classmates. Let's go on the job and into the classroom to see how such proactive environments function.

Consider the Environment

Let's suppose the football coach at Gallaudet is giving a lecture on the opposing team's plays before the big game next week. Or perhaps you and your Deaf coworker are asked to attend a work seminar on the ways businesses can use environmentally friendly technology, including demonstrations of new equipment. Deaf and hearing attendees of any assembly or group meeting need to consider beforehand the purpose of the meeting and the space it will take place in to anticipate Deaf people's need in order to be able to participate fully in the event.

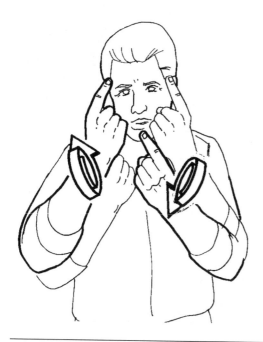

CONSIDER. Remember the formal sign for "think" (on page 40)? "Consider" uses both hands, moving one in a circular clockwise motion and the other in a circular counterclockwise motion. The gears are turning in your head as your brain assesses the challenge at hand to achieve creative solutions.

Consider the Deaf students attending the lecture on football plays at Gallaudet. The students need to be able to see clearly the coach's diagrams on the overhead projector. These diagrams literally "speak for themselves." If the diagrams are drawn carefully and fine points are handwritten legibly on the overhead display, the students can easily focus attention on the visual presentation without the distraction of

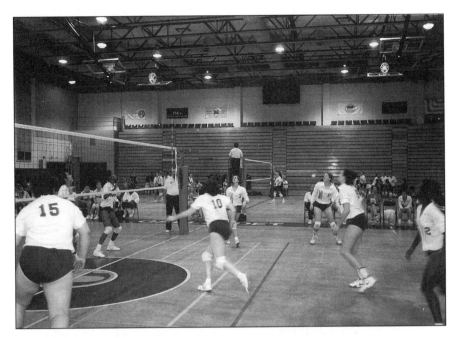

Once on the court, the Gallaudet women's volleyball team and their coach rely on eye contact, natural gesture, and ASL signs to communicate strategies.

having to look constantly from the coach to the overhead display to the playbook. Of course, the lecture hall has been set up so the Deaf students can establish eye contact with the coach and still view the projector screen with no sight-line impediments, and there is enough light retained in the room so the students can see each other in order to communicate. The coach, who is hearing and does not sign, follows each diagrammed play with spoken commentary on its nuances that is signed to the students in ASL through an interpreter. Noticing when several students look down for more than a brief moment to take notes on the lecture, the coach stops speaking until the students look up again and reestablish eye contact. Then, the coach continues on to draw the next play.

Now, let's suppose you and your Deaf coworker are preparing to attend the seminar on environmentally safe business practices. Twenty-five people will be present, and the seminar takes place in a large conference room at your company's headquarters. The seminar sponsors will lecture and demonstrate equipment before holding a question-and-answer session.

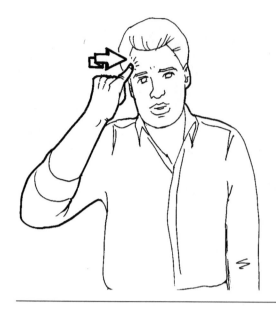

SUPPOSE. In the formal sign for "suppose," or "imagine," the pinky finger of the dominant hand moves outward from the temple, palm facing the body, to show an idea as it runs through your mind and begins to take shape.

Let's make a list of accommodations we need to consider to help make the seminar completely accessible for both Deaf and hearing attendees.

1. Where will people sit? Do they face a lecture podium and demonstration table? Or will attendees be seated in a circle with presenters in the center? Will Deaf participants be able to see the speaker, demonstrator, and interpreter clearly?
2. Has a certified sign language interpreter been provided by your company for the seminar's Deaf attendees, as required by the Americans with Disabilities Act (ADA)? Will the interpreter receive in advance background information on the purpose of the seminar and specialized vocabulary so they can prepare for the event?
3. What light source is required? Will the room be dark or light? Are there windows or blinds behind the speaker that might distract a Deaf person or keep them from establishing eye contact because of excessive glare or brightness?
4. Will a Deaf person be able to establish eye contact with other participants throughout the seminar and during the question-and-answer session? This is especially important if a Deaf person relies on lipreading at any point during the seminar—they

can't get the question, only the answer, if they can't see the other attendees!

We've discovered that work and classroom settings must be "visually friendly" to accommodate the needs of a Deaf person. Deaf and hearing people need to advocate for the best possible conditions to promote good communication. Always ask a Deaf person what is necessary to make an environment acceptable. And don't hesitate to educate coworkers or classmates who may be meeting a Deaf person for the first time. Let them know how easy it is to involve both Deaf and hearing participants successfully in any activity.

The Americans with Disabilities Act (ADA)

The Americans with Disabilities Act (ADA) signed into law by President George Bush in 1990 and fully implemented in 1994, has been called the civil rights act of the disabled. On signing, President Bush stated that ADA would provide America with a new source of workers: "A tremendous pool of people who will bring to jobs diversity, loyalty, proven low turnover rate, and only one request—the chance to prove themselves." The act stipulates that companies and organizations must provide "reasonable accommodation" essential to the successful economic, social, and professional pursuits of qualified individuals with disabilities. For Deaf people, this includes TTYs and telephone relay systems, TV decoders, visible emergency alarms, and other devices that can help facilitate communication in public settings. It also includes the right of Deaf individuals to be provided qualified, certified sign language interpreters. Hiring interpreters is the responsibility of schools, companies, and organizations—not the responsibility of the deaf person!

In a few short years, the ADA has enhanced hearing society's awareness of the services and devices available to connect them with the Deaf community and its talented members. ASL, now recognized as a complete language, is seen by thousands of hearing people across the United States as they attend conferences, theater events, and musical performances where ASL interpreters are present for Deaf attendees; television commercials feature Americans who pitch products to consumers in ASL—everything from cheese to aspirin—with English subtitles. Deaf and hearing communities both benefit from this increased interaction and mutual respect, and our nation's culture grows richer and stronger because of it. President Bill Clinton, in his commencement address to the 1994 graduating class of Gallaudet University said, "The ADA is part of the seamless web of civil rights that so many have worked for so long to build in America, a constant fabric wrapped in the hopes and aspirations of all right-thinking Americans. As your president, I pledge to see that it is fully implemented and aggressively enforced—in schools, in the workplace, in government, in public places. It is time to move from exclusion to inclusion, from dependence to independence, from paternalism to empowerment."

As you meet Deaf people on the job, at school, and in your community always look for new ways to include them in whatever is happening. Ask Deaf people what services or devices they require to make an environment acceptable for proper communication. Add your voice to theirs as an advocate for Deaf rights, and for ASL. Deaf people cannot learn to communicate with hearing people by using their ears. But hearing people *can* learn to communicate with Deaf people by using their eyes and hands to learn sign language. That is what you are doing by using this book!

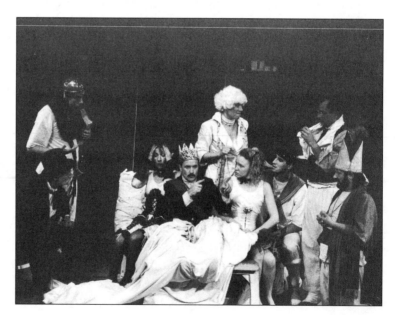

The Gallaudet theater company performs plays in ASL. Theater is a wonderful forum for capturing human emotions and experiences that appeal to both Deaf and hearing audiences. Theaters can provide sign language interpreters for Deaf audience members interested in experiencing plays performed in English.

Communicating through Interpreters

In educational and business settings, qualified sign language interpreters are very effective at facilitating communication between hearing and Deaf consumers. Imagine that a French exchange student who spoke no English came to study at your university, or a Swiss businessperson from your company's international division was transferred to your department here in the United States for a year to study your operating systems, and this person spoke only Italian. Interpreters would be needed so that both English and non-English speakers could be easily understood. The same logic is true for Deaf people who use ASL as their native language. Sign language interpreters are particularly effective in group settings where there is more than one speaker and where constant physical activity or movement can make it difficult for a Deaf person to concentrate visually for long periods of time. Interpreters are also expected to be familiar with any specialized vocabulary (such as medical, legal, or computer terms) needed to communicate efficiently in a variety of situations.

It is a wonderful idea to approach interpreter referral agencies or consulting firms in your area to set up workshops at your school or office designed to teach hearing employees basic sign skills and specialized vocabulary that will help them communicate more effectively with Deaf employees and consumers. A consulting firm can also work with hearing and Deaf employees to set up the most efficient and acceptable environment—from the placement of furnishings to proper lighting and judicious use of electronic devices, such as TTYs (especially effective for a mail-order business with Deaf clients) or e-mail networking.

Remember, however, that individuals with beginning sign language skills are not capable of acting as interpreters and should not be asked to interpret in formal situations. Family members and friends of a Deaf person should be respected as such and also not be asked to interpret; personal relationships may make it hard to stay neutral! Interpreters have a code of ethics that requires them to accurately and objectively relay information between the parties involved without editing or interjecting personal opinions. All conversation is kept strictly confidential.

Dialogue

ASL Gloss

MISS WHAT YOU SAID   INTERPRETER   ME   NEED

Note: Remember, an ASL gloss is only an artificial representation of a three-dimensional language. When signing the dialogue in ASL, remember to use all five of its basic components: (1) eye contact, (2) facial expression, (3) body language, (4) mouth movements, and (5) hand movements.

English Translation

I am missing what you are saying! We need a sign language interpreter.

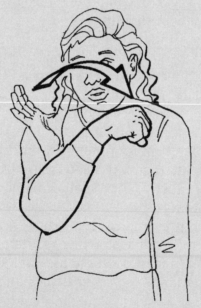

MISS WHAT YOU SAID

Tips for Working with Interpreters

1. Speak plainly and clearly, at normal speed and tone. Speaking slowly or more loudly will not make you better understood and can be viewed by the Deaf person as condescending.

2. Speak directly to the Deaf person, not the interpreter. Avoid saying things like "Tell him" or "Tell her." You want the Deaf person to be actively engaged in the conversation.

3. Interpreters do not edit your remarks. They will translate whatever is said, exactly as it is said. Further, remarks made by any speaker within the presence of the Deaf person will be translated. Avoid the embarrassment of saying something not intended for the Deaf person—for instance, don't inadvertently reveal a surprise party for your Deaf coworker's promotion by announcing it at the end of a meeting!

4. Avoid speaking confidentially to the interpreter, who is present only to translate—not to express opinions or become personally involved in your conversation.

5. Speak one at a time when working with an interpreter—they can sign only for one speaker at a time and are not able to prioritize the importance of various speakers in the room.

6. Ask someone to take notes for the Deaf person while they watch the interpreter. It is hard for the Deaf person to do both at the same time! Remember that meeting or class notes rarely take the place of face-to-face conversation and should not be substituted for a Deaf person's attendance and full participation in discussions and involvement in the decision-making process.

7. Consult the Deaf person about where everyone—the interpreter, and both Deaf and hearing participants, should sit or stand for the most effective placement to facilitate communication.

8. A Deaf person needs time to focus on changes from one speaker to another. Allow for the time lag, often one or two sentences behind, for a Deaf person to contribute to the conversation. The deaf person does have a voice through an interpreter and can participate actively.

At School

Dialogue

ASL Gloss

TEACHER: **HOMEWORK   REMEMBER   YOU**
    [Questioning facial expression: yes/no?]

STUDENT: **EVERY DAY   FORGET ME   NOT**
    [Shake head no]

Note: Remember, an ASL gloss is only an artificial representation of a three-dimensional language. When signing the dialogue in ASL, remember to use all five of its basic components: (1) eye contact, (2) facial expression, (3) body language, (4) mouth movements, and (5) hand movements.

English Translation

TEACHER: Remember to take your homework assignment with you.

STUDENT: I take it with me every day and always do my homework.

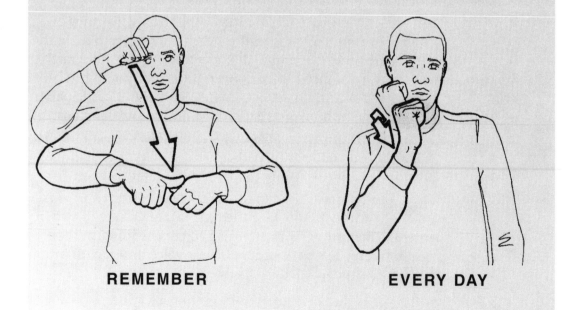

REMEMBER   **EVERY DAY**

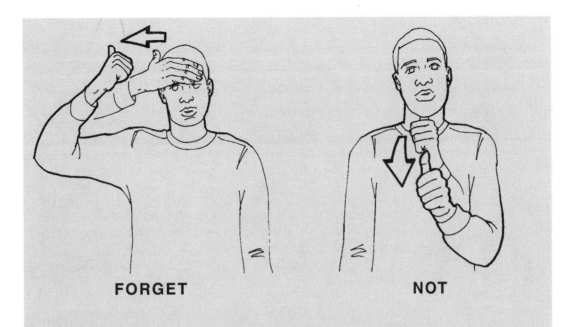

FORGET

NOT

HOMEWORK. Perform the formal signs for "home-work" (on pages 98 and 37).

Dialogue

ASL Gloss

TEACHER: BOOK   ENGLISH   WHERE?   GIVE ME

STUDENT: OVERLOOK

TEACHER: AGAIN?   BOOK OPEN   READ

Note: Remember, an ASL gloss is only an artificial representation of a three-dimensional language. When signing the dialogue in ASL, remember to use all five of its basic components: (1) eye contact, (2) facial expression, (3) body language, (4) mouth movements, and (5) hand movements.

English Translation

TEACHER: Where is your English book? Please give it to me.

STUDENT: Oh, here it is, right in front of me. I didn't even see it.

TEACHER: Again? Open your book and read the assignment.

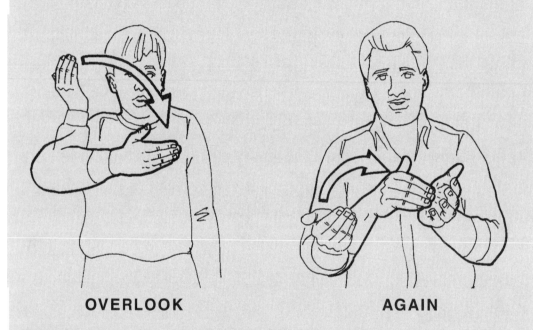

OVERLOOK   **AGAIN**

ENGLISH. Face the nondominant palm to the floor. Rest the dominant palm, also facing the floor, on the wrist of the nondominant hand to represent the hand on the cane or umbrella of an English gentleman.

GIVE. Bring the fingertips and thumb of the dominant hand together, with the palm facing up toward the ceiling. This is a directional verb; the sign moves where the action is intended. For "give me," the sign moves toward the signer; for "give her/him," the sign moves toward the indicated person.

BOOK. Bring the flat five-hands together with palms facing toward the ceiling and pinky fingers touching each other. To "open the book," begin with palms touching and drop them open to the sides as if opening a book. To "close the book," bring the palms back together to touch again.

READ. Extend the middle and index fingers of the dominant hand and place them under the eye, palm facing the body, to touch the middle finger on the cheek; this is "seeing." Then, bring the fingers near the upturned palm of the base hand and move them across the hand to show the eyes "reading" the page.

Directional verbs like "give" and "have" are used in a very concrete way in sign language. "Give the book to her" would be signed

BOOK   GIVE HER

The sign for "give" would move toward "her." You do this without making the formal sign for "her"; we know who is meant from the movement of the sign. Remember that hand movement is one of the four basic elements of formal ASL signs, along with handshape, palm orientation, and placement.

The formal sign for "have" is very similar. For example, the answer to "Where is the book?" is:

TABLE   HAS

This translates into English as "The book is on the table." Notice that the object of the sentence, *book*, is inherent in the ASL answer and does not need to be signed. *Book* has not been left out of the answer; as a concept, it is understood *visually*. To sign the word *book* would be redundant according to the grammatical rules of ASL.

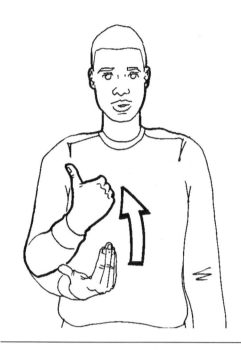

HAVE. This sign for "have" is used strictly in the sense of possessing something and, as above, can apply to inanimate things "having" an object—such as a sweater in a drawer or a vase on a shelf. The sign would not be used to say "I have been" or "Have you ever," because verb tenses are formed differently in ASL, as we have already learned.

On the Job

Dialogue

ASL Gloss

COWORKER #1:
CURIOUS   SUPERVISOR   GO   MEETING   IMPORTANT   ?

COWORKER #2:
HEAR   IMPORTANT   !   *or* HEAR   UNIMPORTANT   !

Note: Remember, an ASL gloss is only an artificial representation of a three-dimensional language. When signing the dialogue in ASL, remember to use all five of its basic components: (1) eye contact, (2) facial expression, (3) body language, (4) mouth movements, and (5) hand movements.

English Translation

COWORKER #1: I am wondering if the meeting the supervisor is attending is an important one?

COWORKER #2: Yes, I heard it is important.   *or*   No, I heard it is not important.

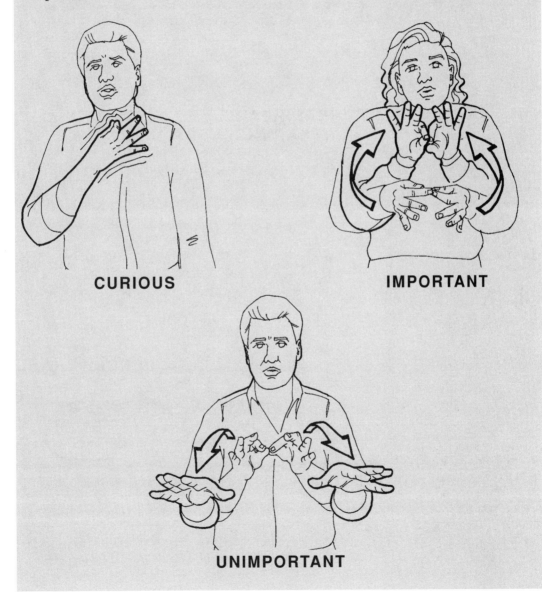

CURIOUS

IMPORTANT

UNIMPORTANT

The formal signs for "important" and "unimportant" move in opposite directions to show opposite meanings.

SUPERVISOR. Place the dominant five-hand on the shoulder, palm facing the floor, as if touching the epaulets of an officer. This is also the formal sign for "coach."

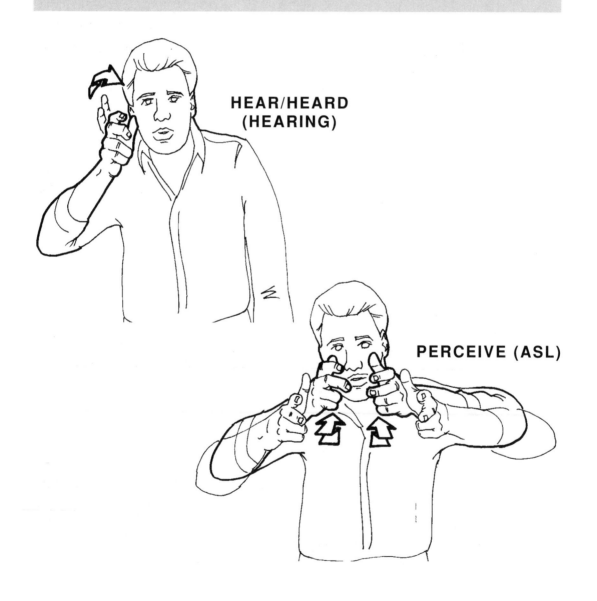

HEAR/HEARD
(HEARING)

PERCEIVE (ASL)

In ASL, there are two signs for "listening": one for Deaf and one for hearing. The sign used in the "At Work" dialogue conveys the meaning that the supervisor is hearing; the supervisor "listens" with their ears. So, the sign moves the index and middle fingers next to the face, toward the ear. ASL, however, is a three-dimensional *visual* language. A Deaf supervisor receives information, or "hears," by looking and perceiving with their *eyes*. So, the sign for receiving information through ASL, "perceive," is performed using both hands, with the index and middle fingers moving toward the eyes, and the placement in front of the face. Communication enters the eyes, not the ears. This important distinction shows in which language a Deaf or hearing person received a message—English or ASL.

We've learned that collaboration between Deaf and hearing is essential on the job and at school to create dynamic and creative environments with maximum access to communication available for all participants! We also understand the importance of advocating for the use of ASL in office, classroom, and community settings, for full implementation of the ADA regulations. In the next chapter, we go outdoors with our Deaf friends to discover how ASL is used when getting around.

EXERCISES

These exercises are designed to help you in real-world interactions with Deaf people at school and on the job. See how bold and innovative you can be in coming up with new and effective ways to collaborate on work and school projects!

Chat Room

Just like on-line services, create a "chat room" of your own to compare ideas about how to improve the classroom or workplace for Deaf and hearing coworkers and to learn new signs and practice ASL. Arrange a weekly time and place to meet with hearing and Deaf classmates or coworkers. Use this time to discuss situations, procedures, etiquette,

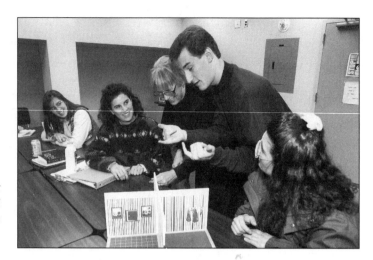

A Gallaudet professor and students discuss a class project.

and vocabulary. Ask the Deaf person for advice on the best signs to use to get the precise meaning in ASL. Invite supervisors to attend so they can get a good picture of what is happening and what the concerns of students, teachers, or employees really are. Invite a sign language interpreter to conduct a workshop on the most effective ways to procure and work with interpreters; invite a Deaf person to conduct a workshop on ASL.

If there are no Deaf people in your class or workplace, make a list of all the things in your environment that might help or hinder communication with a Deaf person. Which ones are solved by recent advances in technology? What might people have done before the new advances in computer and telecommunications came about to accomplish the same results?

Working Together

In your class, or at your workplace, design a project where hearing and Deaf classmates and coworkers collaborate closely. Establish a time frame and clearly indicate the assignments of each group member. Keep a journal of the project's progress, including any problems the group encounters in communication, and how they are solved. When the project is completed, give a bilingual presentation, in English and ASL, at your school and office. Invite people from other classes or departments to attend. Let them see for themselves how successful teamwork between Deaf and hearing can be!

Additional Vocabulary

COMPUTER. Extend the nondominant arm and hand in front of you to form a base, palm facing the floor. With the dominant hand in the "C" or "claw" handshape, touch the pinky to the base arm and move it toward the elbow to show the act of compiling data.

DESK. See "table" on page 24.

EMPLOYEE. Perform the sign for "work" (on page 37). Then, place both hands in the flat five-hand handshape, fingers together, with palms facing toward each other. Move the hands down the sides of the body to show a person.

FILE. To sign the verb "to file" place the nondominant five-hand in front of the body, fingers spread apart and pointing away from you. Move the closed five-hand of the dominant hand, pinky finger facing the open fingers of the nondominant hand, into the spaces between the fingers. You are showing the act of "filing." To sign the noun "file" place the dominant closed five-hand between the index and middle fingers of the nondominant five-hand.

INFORM/NEWS. Bring the fingers and thumb of both hands together and touch the fingertips to the forehead; see "teach/learn" on page 30. Move the hands away from the body, opening the fingers in front of you to disseminate information.

ITEMS/ITEMIZE. Extend the nondominant five-hand in front of the body, fingers spread and pointing away from you. Use the index finger of the dominant hand to touch the fingertips of the base. You are pointing out each element.

LETTER. The thumb of the dominant hand extends from the fist. Move the thumb from about mouth height to touch the thumb of the nondominant hand. The nondominant hand is held in front of the body in a fist with the thumb extended up. It is as if you were licking and placing a stamp on an envelope. This is also the sign used for the noun "mail."

OFFICE. See "room" on page 30. Or perform the signs for "work- room" (see "work" on page 37).

PHOTOCOPY. Extend the nondominant arm and hand in front of you to form a base, palm facing the floor. Touch the fingertips, spread in the open five-hand, of the dominant hand to the palm of the base hand. Move the fingers in a downward motion to bring the fingertips and thumb together, as if you are pulling copies from the machine. For small numbers of copies (less than five) repeat the motion to show how many copies are made. Or perform the motion one time and then sign the number: "copy-1," for example.

PRINT/PRINTOUT. To sign "print," as in "newspaper" or "printed word," place the nondominant flat five-hand in front of the body, fingers together and palm facing up. Rest the thumb of the dominant hand on the base palm and tap the forefinger onto the thumb, as if putting a letter down onto the page or pressing down a character key on a computer keyboard. To sign "printout," place both hands in front of the body, one palm facing down and one up, with fingers spread. Bend the thumbs into the wrist. Together, move the hands from left to right and repeat the motion. You are showing the flow of the paper as it comes out of the computer printer.

TYPE/INPUT DATA. Use both hands and mime the motion of typing on a keyboard. The hands remain stationary while the fingers move as if typing on a keyboard. It's natural gesture!

WHAT. Open both five-hands, palms up, in front of the body. Elbows are bent and shoulders are slightly raised. This is also a natural sign.

Chapter 8

Getting Around

American Sign Language (ASL) is the perfect language to use when getting around. Imagine we are visiting New York City and set off on a tour of the United Nations building with a diverse group of people from many different countries, each speaking a different language. How do we ask questions, give or understand directions, and communicate among ourselves or with the tour guide? Think about the five basic components of ASL: (1) eye contact, (2) facial expression, (3) body language, (4) mouth movements, and (5) hand movements. Communicating with our eyes, bodies, faces, and hands, we are able to give and receive information using the three-dimensional concepts of sign language. We communicate without English or foreign words. Sign language is the universal human language!

Now, instead of the United Nations, picture the Deaf Way Conference, a landmark gathering of Deaf communities and organizations from around the world, sponsored by Gallaudet University and held in Washington, D.C. Here, we rely on *Gestuno*—an international sign language that embodies the expressive creativity of natural gesture—as we make new friends, enjoy sharing our similarities and differences with

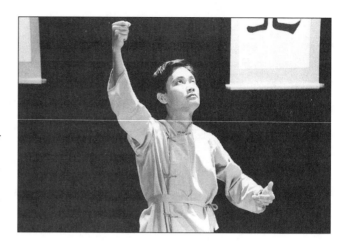

Gestuno is a gestural form of communication used at international Deaf events and meetings.

each other, and participate in Deaf Way's celebration of cooperation between cultures.

Let Your Fingers Do the Walking

American Sign Language makes efficient use of gestures to describe, in just a matter of seconds, how two people interact with each other. It is done with a minimum of effort, and in a way anybody can understand—whether they know sign language or are English speaking. You'll find you can tell the story of an entire situation. Let's begin by recalling the formal ASL sign for "meet" (on page 42).

MEET. Hold both hands in front of the body with the pointer fingers extended up toward the ceiling and the fingers touching the palms. Palms face each other. Move the hands together so that the meat of the palm touches the meat of the palm. Two people meet.

Already, you are using your pointer fingers to show two people moving toward each other. But that's just the beginning. How do the people feel about each other? Are they in a hurry or late? Are they glad to see each other? What happens when they come together? We will use our bodies, faces, and hands to communicate all of this vital information. In these movements, both hands are considered dominant, as each provides meaning necessary for a complete understanding of what is signed. So, look at both of the signer's hands simultaneously. Also take careful note of the signer's facial expressions and body language; they will provide essential clues about the nature of the action as it unfolds.

Let's take a look at several different scenarios. What happens between the people in each one?

1. Place the left pointer finger in a stationary position in front of your body. The right pointer finger races in quickly to meet it, shaking nervously as it moves. The signer uses a wide-eyed facial expression and blinks, swallowing hard. The approaching person is anxious because they are late for the meeting. When the fingers come together, the signer's facial expression turns to one of dismay as the focus shifts to the left pointer finger. Simultaneously, the left hand turns the finger away from the body and the signer's head turns with it to show the displeasure of the waiting person as they turn to walk away.

2. Bring the pointer fingers together so they touch at the sides with the palms facing out from the body. Move the fingers and arms apart; turn the fingers out as the arms extend from your sides. The people are moving in opposite directions. This is also used to represent the English idioms "We went our separate ways" and "We grew apart naturally."

3. Hold the pointer fingers at either side of the body. Move them across the body so that each finger is now positioned on the opposite side. The fingers literally move past each other: "We just missed each other."

4. The index and middle fingers extended and pointing toward two people is a versatile sign. With the palm facing up, this sign means "you and me," "the two of us," "the two of them," or "you two."

5. The open five-hand, thumb facing the body, moves directly to touch the extended pointer finger, palm facing out, of the other hand. The spread fingers wave back and forth. The signer smiles: "You are a popular person."

In each of these situations, the pointer fingers are *descriptors*, handshapes used to describe specific people as they move or perform an action. The signer uses facial expressions and body language to convey the adjectives and adverbs that enrich the situation's context. To indicate a particular gender, a signer performs the sign for "man" to identify one pointer finger and "woman" to identify the other. That finger then represents the appropriate person throughout the ASL conversation.

Storytellers call creating situations like the ones above, establishing dramatic situations, because they set the action and reveal how the characters feel. How many situations can you create in ASL? Try practicing with these:

- One person snubs the other unwittingly, then follows after to apologize.
- Two people notice each other for the first time, peeking timidly at first, then growing bolder until they work up the courage to meet.
- One person is lost and frightened. The other searches for and finds them, with great relief. Both are happy.
- We haven't seen each other in a long time. We were surprised to bump into each other.
- Imagine two lovers running toward each other through a field of flowers. How would they move?

Everything you do with your eyes, faces, bodies, and hands adds meaning to the story you paint with ASL pictures. Let your imagination lead you to become as uninhibited as possible, as you have fun communicating dramatic situations to others in sign language.

Asking Questions

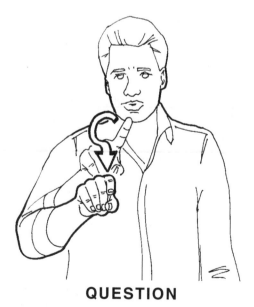

QUESTION

QUESTION. To keep from getting lost, we ask questions. Hopefully, the person we ask will give us clear directions to reach our destination. You can turn any ASL statement into a question by performing the formal sign for "question" at the end of the thought. Therefore, "Turn left at the next corner" becomes "Turn left at the next corner?" when the sign for "question" is added.

When giving and receiving directions, feel free to make use of natural gestures. Point to the left or right, up or down. Count subway stops on your fingers. Wind your flat five-hand in the direction the road will take. Make the flat five-hand into a wall, palm facing out, and use the extended pointer finger to show a person walking up to it and turning the corner. Use the body as if it is a compass to indicate north, south, east, and west. In front of a mirror, or with a partner, give directions to these common places: (1) school, (2) the library, (3) the grocery store, (4) your house, (5) a friend or relative's house.

DIRECTIONS. With both open five-hands, touch the thumb and forefinger together; this is the signed letter "F." Face the palms toward each other. In front of the body, move the hands alternately forward and backward in straight lines. The base meaning of this sign is "explain." It can also be used to show "instructions."

A signer can be even more specific when asking a question by using their facial expression to show that a yes-or-no answer is required.

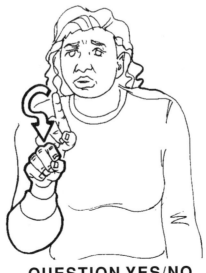

QUESTION YES/NO

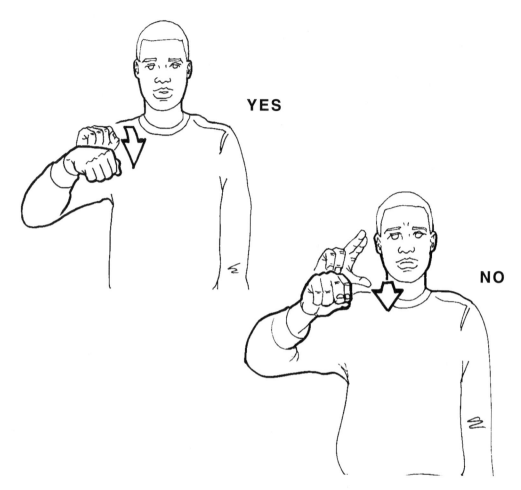

YES

NO

   The gestural nature of these signs makes them easy for both signers and nonsigners to understand. Nodding the head yes or shaking it no appropriately, with a look of approval or disapproval on the face, enhances the universal message. For instance, you take your lunch break at a local restaurant with your Deaf coworker. As you sit down at the counter, your Deaf coworker proceeds to get the attention of the waitperson by waving a hand politely in the air. Using a combination of natural gesture and formal sign, your coworker orders. First, they point to the entry for Chef Salad on the menu; and then, with a questioning expression, they bring the thumb and forefinger together to show "small," followed by the formal sign for "question." The waitperson holds up a small-sized bowl and your coworker nods yes. Types of soda are not specified on the menu, so your coworker points to the soda fountain. Point, point, point to the third item, root beer. The waitperson touches a different soda sign tentatively and your coworker shakes their head no, and points again. Success: Root beer. This is basic communication, easily achieved.

Why? Why? Why?

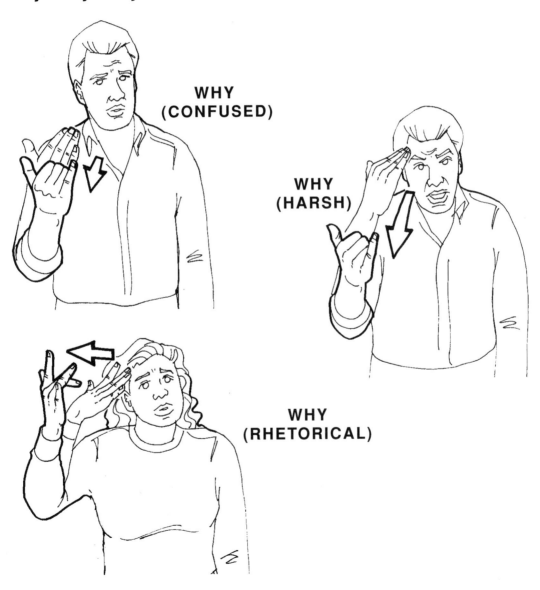

WHY
(CONFUSED)

WHY
(HARSH)

WHY
(RHETORICAL)

Sometimes, we need more than a simple yes-or-no answer; we need to know "why." In spoken English, the way a question is said out loud, the tone of voice, conveys a deeper meaning. As we have already learned, the formal elements of ASL signs and the basic components of ASL accomplish the same enhancement of meaning. All three illustrations for "why" use the same basic handshape. In the first, a confused facial expression shows that the signer does not fully understand: "Turn left at the next corner? Why do I want to do that?" In the second, a swift and sharply downward hand movement, combined with a harsh facial expression, shows disbelief or disapproval: "Turn left at the next corner? Why should I?" The third illustration shows the decision-making yes-and-no process and is used to reply to the original question: "Turn left at the next corner. Why? To avoid traffic." The rhetorical "why" functions in ASL the same way the word *because* functions in spoken and written English. *Because* is a very English construction; it is an abstract concept without an easily visible picture. In sign language, *because* is usually avoided in favor of the naturally expressive rhetorical "why."

Getting Around

Dialogue

ASL Gloss

FRIEND #1: DRIVE MALL WHY (Rhetorical) SHIRT ME BUY. WHAT DO YOU ?

FRIEND #2: DO/DO/DO PRESENTATION. DINNER MEET TWO OF US ?

FRIEND #1: SURE TIME SEVEN ?

FRIEND #2: SURE

Note: Remember, an ASL gloss is only an artificial representation of a three-dimensional language. When signing the dialogue in ASL, remember to use all five of its basic components: (1) eye contact, (2) facial expression, (3) body language, (4) mouth movements, and (5) hand movements.

English Translation

FRIEND #1: I am driving to the mall because I want to buy a new shirt. What are you doing?

FRIEND #2: I am busy working on my presentation. Let's meet for dinner.

FRIEND #1: Sure. How about seven tonight?

FRIEND #2: Okay.

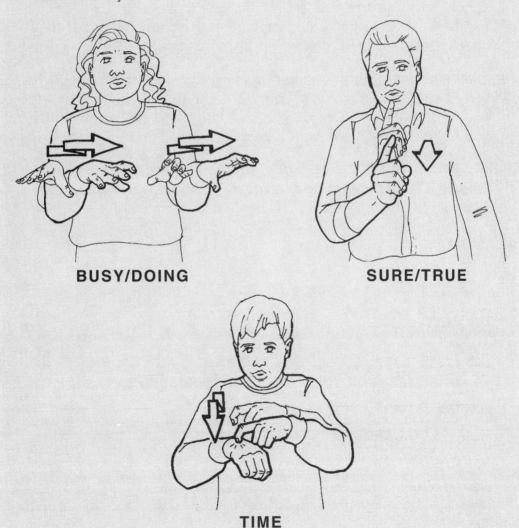

BUSY/DOING

SURE/TRUE

TIME

As we've already learned, the sign "what do?" is used to ask the question, "What are you doing?" or "What do you want to do?" You can also use it to say, "What can I do about the situation?" The sign for "busy/doing," however, is used to show the physical *act* of doing something. It can be linked with any verb to show you are very busy or to show continued activity.

DRIVE/CAR. Picture an imaginary steering wheel in front of you. Take your hands and grip the wheel, closing your hands into fists. Move the hands back and forth in a steering motion. For "bus" or "truck," move the hands farther apart to show a bigger steering wheel.

SHOPPING/MALL. Bring the thumb and fingers of the dominant hand together, palm facing up, and rest it on the upturned palm of the base hand. This is the formal sign for "money." To "buy," slide the dominant hand along the palm one time. For "shopping/mall" repeat the motion: "buy, buy, buy."

PRESENTATION/SPEECH/LECTURE. Wave the dominant five-hand briskly in the air like Queen Elizabeth acknowledging a crowd.

Dialogue

ASL Gloss

MOTHER: SISTER   BICYCLE   COLOR   FEEL   SHE   WANT   ?

SON: DON'T CARE

MOTHER: LOOK AROUND   MAYBE   WANT   BLUE

SON: GREEN   ME   WANT

Note: Remember, an ASL gloss is only an artificial representation of a three-dimensional language. When signing the dialogue in ASL, remember to use all five of its basic components: (1) eye contact, (2) facial expression, (3) body language, (4) mouth movements, and (5) hand movements.

English Translation

MOTHER: What color bicycle do you think your sister would like to have?

SON: I don't care what color she wants.

MOTHER: Let's see what they have. Maybe she'll want a blue one.

SON: I want a green bicycle.

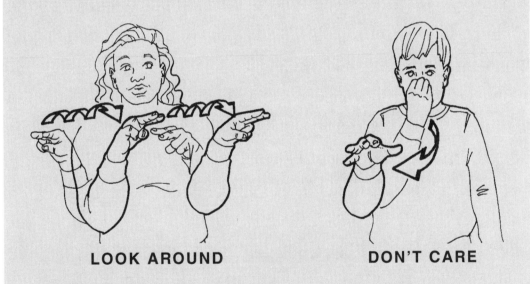

LOOK AROUND   **DON'T CARE**

COLOR. The dominant open five-hand, fingers spread apart, palm facing the body, is placed so the index and middle fingers touch the chin just below the lips, moving back and forth in front of the chin.

BLUE. Take the flat five-hand and hold it up, palm facing out. Fold the thumb into the palm. This is the signed letter "B." Shake the hand in the air to show "blue."

GREEN. With the dominant hand, make a fist with the thumb facing toward the ceiling. Then, extend the index finger across the body, so the palm turns toward you. This is the signed letter "G." Shake the hand in the air to show "green."

BICYCLE. The fists of each hand move in an alternating circular motion away from the body, palms face down. Your hands are the moving pedals of a bike.

MAYBE. With both hands, make fists and extend the thumbs into the air. Line up the knuckles and move the hands alternately up and down in front of the body. Things could go "either way."

Politeness Counts

When getting around, we want to be careful to acknowledge someone who helps us find our way. In Deaf culture, "Please," "Thank you," "You're welcome," and "I'm sorry" are usually shown on the face. The facial expression says it all. Deaf people tend to use the formal signs for these concepts when conversing with hearing people, or when they are in a very formal situation. Usually, a smile is all that is needed to say "Thank you" or "You're welcome." Deaf people will often use the sign "sure/true" with the meaning, "You're welcome," when signing informally. A considerate expression asks a polite "Please," while a heartfelt expression conveys sincere personal regrets.

As in any community, Deaf or hearing, the most important thing to remember is this: always show

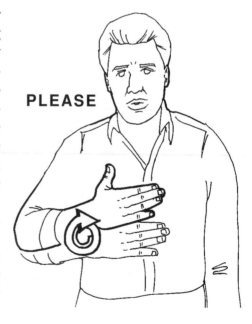

PLEASE

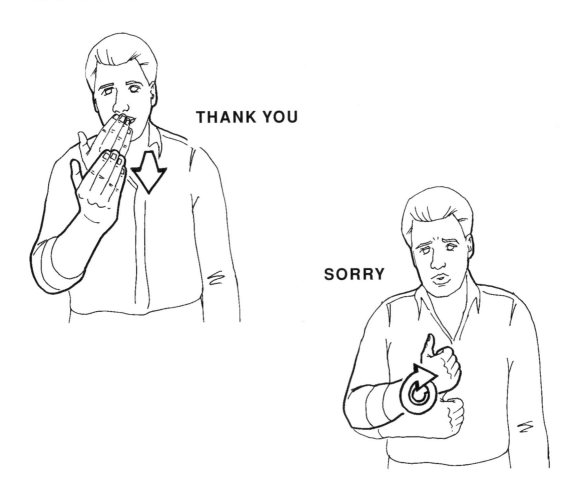

THANK YOU

SORRY

the proper respect to others. When communicating in ASL, be sure to hold eye contact until all parties have exchanged courtesies.

YOU'RE WELCOME. Using the flat five-hand, palm upturned with the thumb facing out, bring the hand toward you in a sweeping motion and nod the head as if taking a bow!

In this chapter, we've seen firsthand how easy it is to get around using American Sign Language. In fact, using our eyes, faces, bodies, and hands, we can ask for and receive directions and information quickly and efficiently. In the next chapter, we'll explore the concepts of past, present, and future, to learn how to add the dimension of time to our movements. See you there!

EXERCISE

Use this exercise to have fun as you paint sign language pictures to visit exotic places and show how to get there.

Travel Agency

With a partner, or in a group, write down on individual pieces of paper the names of places all over the globe where you and your friends might imagine taking exciting vacations. Be adventurous. Fold the papers and place them in a bowl. Each person chooses a place from the bowl and begins to describe the ultimate vacation experience to the travel agent.

1. Show where the place is located on a map and how near or far away it might be. What mode of transportation will you use to travel to your vacation spot?
2. What does the place look like?
3. How do the native people of your vacation paradise dress? What are their local customs?
4. What is the weather like?
5. What kind of cuisine is served?
6. Are there landmarks or special places at your vacation spot that you'll be visiting? Describe their appearance and function.
7. What kinds of souvenirs will you want to bring home?
8. What activities will you enjoy on your vacation?

Give full reign to your sense of playfulness and imagination as your sign language travels take you around the globe—and, who knows, maybe to the moon and beyond the stars!

Additional Vocabulary

AIRPLANE. With the dominant five-hand, palm facing the floor, extend the thumb and pinky finger to represent the wings of a plane; draw the other fingers into the palm. Using the back of the base hand as a landing strip, touch the "airplane" lightly to it and "take off," moving the hand up into the air.

BEACH. Place your nondominant hand, palm facing down and arm extended, in front of you to represent the beach. With the dominant open five-hand, brush the fingers back and forth over the beach; bend the wrist to show waves breaking against the sand.

BOAT. Cup your hands together to form the hull of a boat. Move the hands up and out from the body to show the boat sailing over the waves.

CHARGE ON CREDIT. Place your fist, thumb facing toward the ceiling, on the upturned palm of the flat base hand. Drag the fist across the palm to represent the motion of putting a credit card into a receipt-stamping machine.

CITY. Touch your fingertips together to represent the roof of a house. Repeat the motion to show many houses.

COLD. Hold both fists in front of the body and shake them in toward each other as if you are shivering from the cold.

HOT. Hold the dominant hand, in the "C" or "claw" handshape, just below your mouth, palm facing the body. Push the palm down and away as if moving a hot beverage away from your lips.

LIBRARY. Extend the forefinger and thumb of the dominant hand, palm facing out; draw the other fingers into the palm. This is the signed letter "L." Shake the hand slightly back and forth in the air in front of you.

PARIS. Extend the pointer and middle fingers of both hands as you sweep them in an upward motion to touch the fingertips together—as if to make an Eiffel Tower in the air.

RAIN. Using both hands in the "C" or "claw" handshape, palms facing downward, move the hands in a repeated downward motion. The intensity of the motion shows the severity of the storm: A light rain falls slowly and delicately; heavy rain falls fast and forcefully.

ROAD. Use both five-hands, fingers closed together, to make a road or path in front of your body.

SNOW. Using both hands in the open five-hand, palms facing out and arms extended in front of your body, wiggle the fingers while moving your hands down to represent snowflakes falling.

SUBWAY. With the dominant five-hand, palm facing the floor, extend the thumb and pinky finger and draw the other fingers into the palm. Place the nondominant hand and arm in front of the body, palm also facing the floor, and run the dominant hand back and forth under the "tracks."

TRAVEL/TRIP. Crook the index and middle fingers of the dominant hand, palm facing down; draw the other fingers and thumb into the palm. Swing the hand in a motion away from the body to show the motion of traveling.

VACATION. Using both open five-hands, touch the thumbs to both sides of the upper chest. Imagine you are wearing overalls and tucking your thumbs into them in a stance representing a break from your work.

WIND. Using both open five-hands, sweep the hands from side to side, slightly below the chin. As they sweep, turn the wrists so that one palm faces the body while the other faces away. This represents the blowing breeze.

Chapter 9

What Time Is It?

American Sign Language (ASL) is a language we see. When we communicate in sign, we send a message with our bodies, faces, and hands that is understood visually. The message exists in space; it is three-dimensional. The three dimensions make sign language an active language that paints pictures of events as they unfold. How do these events find their place in time? How do we know when something happens?

Time in Three Dimensions

In sign language, the abstract concepts of past, present, and future are represented by the body. Your body becomes the physical center of time: the present moment. The space in front of your body represents the future. The space behind your body represents the past. Let's look at the formal ASL signs for "future," "present," and "past."

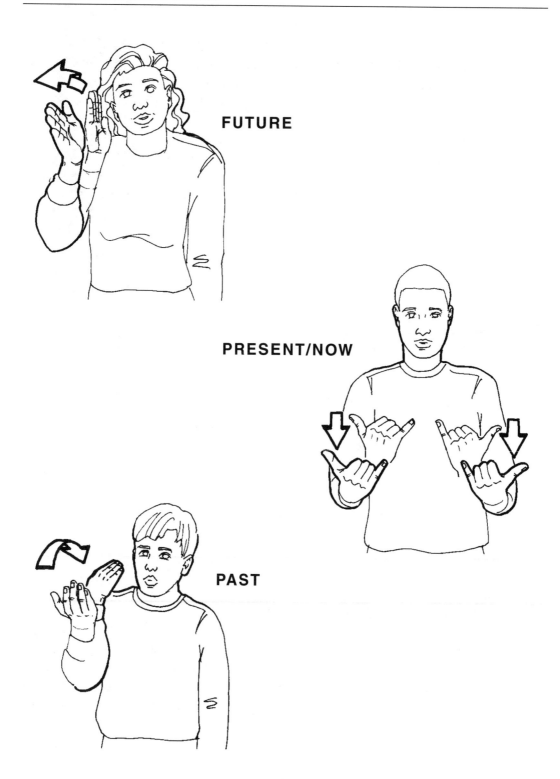

FUTURE

PRESENT/NOW

PAST

These signs, deeply rooted in natural gesture, show us where the body is within the timeline we create with our bodies in space. The future is before us, yet to be seen; the hand moves outward from the eyes. The present is with us, here and now; the hands move in a downward motion along the body. The past is behind us, already seen and processed; the hand moves over the shoulder, past the eyes. How do you show an event that will take place far in the future? It's easy, extend the arm before you in a long motion. To show something that happened a long time ago, make a broad motion over your shoulder. In the expressive and immediate context of sign language, a language that moves in three dimensions, time flows from the body in an arc that represents a lifetime of experience.

The formal ASL signs for "tomorrow," "today," and yesterday," also follow the arc of your body's timeline.

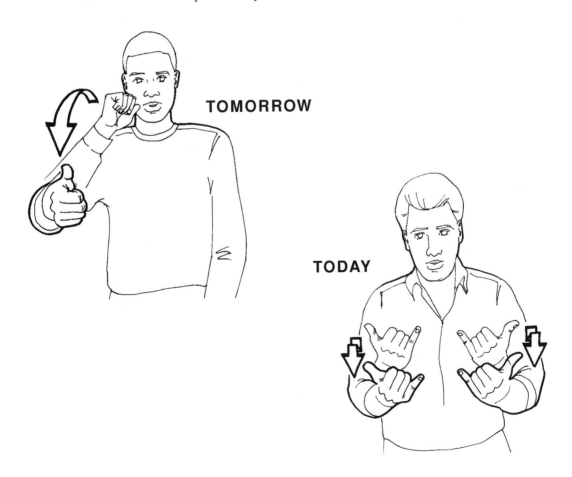

TOMORROW

TODAY

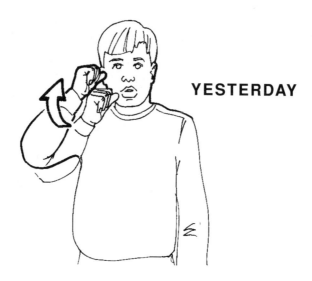

YESTERDAY

Tomorrow is ahead of us, propelling our body forward to meet the future. Today shows what is happening now, on this day; the signs for "present/now" and "today" are almost the same, except that the movement for "today" adds a small bounce of the hands at the base of the motion. "Yesterday" uses the same handshape and palm orientation as the formal sign for "tomorrow," but with the one all-important difference! The hand movement reverses the motion. Where "tomorrow" unwinds to reveal events not yet encountered, "yesterday" rewinds them. Yesterday's events have already been experienced.

It's All in a Day

Let's review the signs for "morning," "noon," and "night." In Chapter 6, we learned that these signs are performed in combination with the formal sign for "eat/food" to denote mealtimes.

"Morning" shows the sun rising. "Noon" shows the sun at its high point, and also evokes the clock's hands pointing straight up at 12:00, or high noon. "Night" shows the sun setting on the horizon. Once again, time, an abstract concept, is made a concrete visual event. Here, it is linked to the experience of watching the sun rise at the start of day and watching it set at day's end (see "sunrise/sunset" on page 30). By

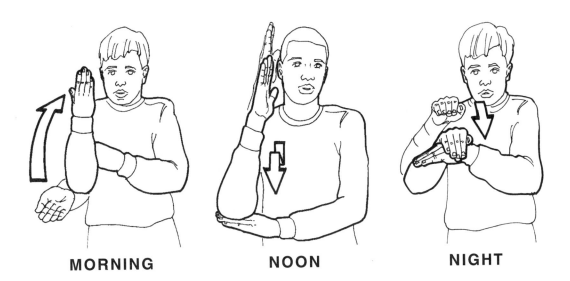

MORNING   **NOON**   **NIGHT**

incorporating these pictures into the formal signs for "breakfast" ("morning-eat/food"), for "lunch" ("noon-eat/food"), and for "dinner" ("night-eat/food"), even mealtimes are placed within the visual context through which we experience the time of day. In sign language, we express the passage of a day in terms of the way we *see* it with our eyes.

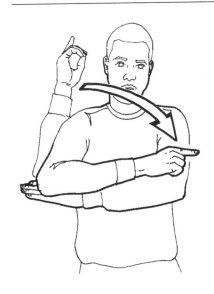

DAY. A day passes in a line of experience that moves from the moment of sunup to the moment of sundown. The handshape for this formal sign is the signed letter "D." Just as our bodies move through time and space, away from our past and forward to our future, they also move through a day's events. Here are some examples.

ENGLISH TRANSLATION: *I worked all day.*

ASL GLOSS:

ME   WORK/WORK/WORK   TODAY

By repeating the sign for "work" (on page 37), followed by the sign for "today," you are communicating that you kept working all day long, or "I worked all day."

ENGLISH TRANSLATION: *Will you do the presentation?*

ASL GLOSS: YOU   PRESENTATION   FUTURE   YOU   ?

The sign for "future" indicates that the presentation takes place at some unspecified future time. You could give the presentation five minutes from now or five days from now. No specific time frame is established.

ENGLISH TRANSLATION: *Will you work on the presentation tomorrow?*

ASL GLOSS: YOU   TOMORROW   WORK   ?
WHAT-DO   PRESENTATION.

In the English sentence and ASL gloss above, we've designated a specific time frame within which the work will take place.

ENGLISH TRANSLATION: *I was awake all night long.*

ASL GLOSS: ME   AWAKE   ALL NIGHT

AWAKE. With both "C"-hands, fingers together, place both hands in front of the eyes to show the big circles of owl eyes. Your eyes are wide open; you are wide awake. This is also the sign for the noun "insomnia."

ALL NIGHT. Begin at the starting point of the sign for "day," except that the handshape changes to the closed five-hand. The five-hand comes out in front of the body, palm facing down, and scoops downward below the base arm. At the bottom of the motion, turn the palm upward to face the base elbow. You are showing the sun revolving all night before coming up in the morning.

Telling Time

Picture yourself in the busy atmosphere of a crowded party scene. It's time to go, and you wave to your friends across the room to get their attention: "Let's leave in five minutes." You point to your watch and hold up five fingers. Yes! Whether the party-goers are Deaf or hearing, the message is communicated simply and effectively through natural gesture. These natural gestures are also the formal manner of expressing clock time in American Sign Language.

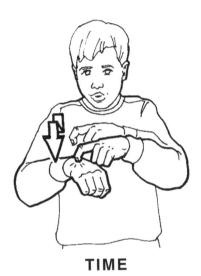

TIME

So, one o'clock = "time-1" (index finger), two o'clock = "time-2" (index and middle fingers), three o'clock = "time-3" (thumb, index, and middle fingers), four o'clock = "time-4" (fingers extended and thumb drawn to palm, five o'clock = "time-5" (thumb and fingers), and so on.

You may use these signs only to show what time it is on the clock. To say how many times something happened, a different combination of signs is used:

ENGLISH TRANSLATION: *I did that work three times.*

ASL GLOSS: WORK　　3　　AGAIN

To help you remember how to sign these two different senses of the concept, "time," correctly, think about the *picture* you are communicating. "Three o'clock" brings to mind the image of a clock face. "Three times" brings to mind the image of a repeated motion or activity.

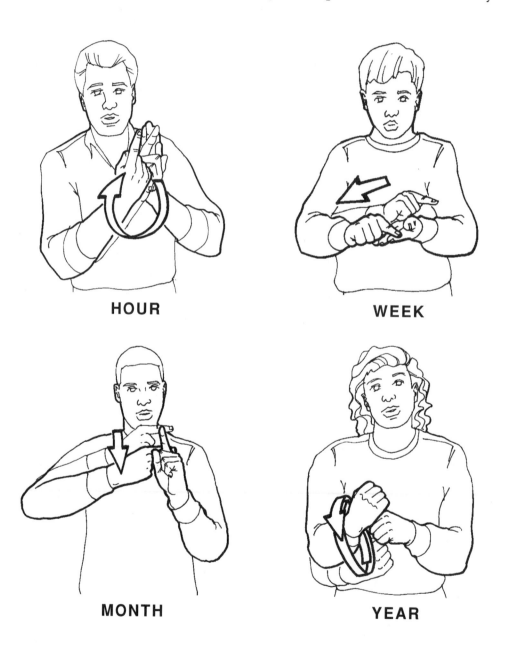

HOUR

WEEK

MONTH

YEAR

HOUR. The formal sign for "hour" uses the base hand as the face of the clock. The index finger of the dominant hand, always pointing straight up, revolves over the base hand in a clockwise motion. To sign "one half hour," the index finger moves only halfway around the clock circle, from the fingertips to the wrist of the base hand.

WEEK. The upturned palm of the base hand now represents a calendar or date book. The extended pointer finger moves across the palm to show the passage of time from Monday through Friday. To sign "every week," repeat the sign for "week" several times; this means "weekly." To sign "two weeks," however, move the index and middle fingers across the palm—this is the signed number "two." For "three weeks," the thumb, index, and middle fingers move across the palm—the dominant hand uses the number sign for "three" to show "three weeks." Now, how do you say "three weeks from now?" or "three weeks ago?" Remember our time line of past, present, and future! "Three weeks from now" begins the motion at the at the wrist of the base palm and continues it forward beyond the fingertips out into the future. "Three weeks ago" takes the motion from a spot just beyond the fingertips and moves it backward over the shoulder of the dominant hand.

MONTH. The dominant extended pointer finger moves in a downward motion from the fingertip to the knuckle of the base finger to show the passage of days in a month. To sign "one month ago," perform the sign for "month" and then "past." "Two months from now" would be "two-month-future."

YEAR. The fists go around each other to show the orbiting motion of the Earth around the sun. The circulating hand is the dominant one. To sign "three years," take the signed number "three" on the dominant hand and revolve it one time around the base. To sign "three years from now," continue the motion by touching the base hand and moving the dominant hand out in front of the body. To sign "three years ago," continue the motion by moving the dominant hand back over the shoulder.

Actions on a Timeline

Just as the body functions as the center for the time flowing between past, present, and future, the three dimensionality of sign language also uses the body to show when actions are performed. In the linear syntax of written and spoken English, time—past, present, and future—is indicated through verb tense. The tense immediately communicates the time frame of the action. But sign language moves in three dimensions and is an active, spatial language. So to understand the timing of an action or event in ASL, we must *see* the time it occurred. Let's look at three more important signs that show when things happen:

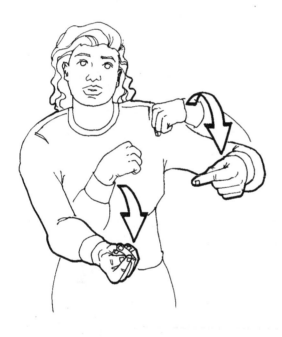

SINCE (TIME). This sign moves outward from the shoulder to indicate a time span that defines when a specific action or event took place. It is used to show "since" only in the sense of a finite amount of time that has passed. For example, in answer to the question, "How long have you been learning sign?," you sign in response: "since-three-year." The English translation is "I've been learning sign language for three years."

In English, the word *since* is often interchanged with the word *because*. As we've already learned, "because" is expressed in sign language by using the formal sign for "why (rhetorical)" (on page 127). "Since" and "because" represent completely different concepts in sign language! To remember the difference between them, think of the visual, or how these concepts *look*. "Since" brings to mind the picture of a timeline, something that has occurred. "Because" brings to mind the yes-and-no process of making decisions, of choosing something.

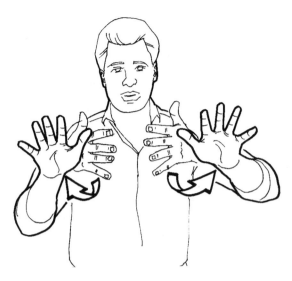

FINISH. The formal sign for "finish" is a very important one in the grammatical structure of sign language; it has several meanings and is used in a much broader context than the English word *finish*. The three primary meanings of the formal sign for "finish" are (1) to denote an action that is completed, (2) to say "that's enough," and (3) to convey the English word "already."

1. Completed action

    ENGLISH TRANSLATION: Friend #1: *Have you eaten?*

    Friend #2: *Yes.*

    ASL GLOSS: Friend #1: EAT   FINISH   YOU   ?

    Friend #2: FINISH

    "Yes" and "no" are not specific enough answers in sign language to *see* the completed action. Performing the sign for "finish" clearly indicates that the action has occurred; you have eaten.

2. Enough

    ENGLISH TRANSLATION: *That's enough work for today.*

    ASL GLOSS: WORK   FINISH   TODAY

    "Finish" can also be signed with the meaning "cut it out" or "that's enough." For example, if someone is making you laugh so hard your stomach hurts, sign "finish" to get them to "cut it out!"

3. Already

ENGLISH TRANSLATION: *I already studied that book.*

ASL GLOSS: ME   BOOK   STUDY   FINISH

By signing "finish" you communicate that you've read the book; you don't need to read it again.

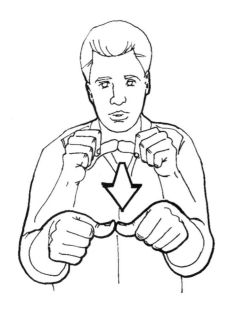

CONTINUE. This sign moves in front of the body to show an action that is still occurring. The action pulls us into the future. For example, the ASL gloss for "I'm still learning" is

ME   LEARN   CONTINUE

Moving in Time

The concept of time is essential to forming complete thoughts in sign language. In order to know when something happens, we need to *see* what time it happens. Representing time in picture form is what establishes verb tenses in ASL. Remember that conversing in sign language is an active experience where both concrete and abstract concepts are shown and understood in three-dimensional pictures. Everything is communicated through our feelings and our bodies.

Translate these English sentences into ASL. Use all of the basic components: (1) eye contact, (2) facial expression, (3) body language,

(4) mouth movements, and (5) hand movements, to make your message as rich in detail as possible. How would you use these new signs:

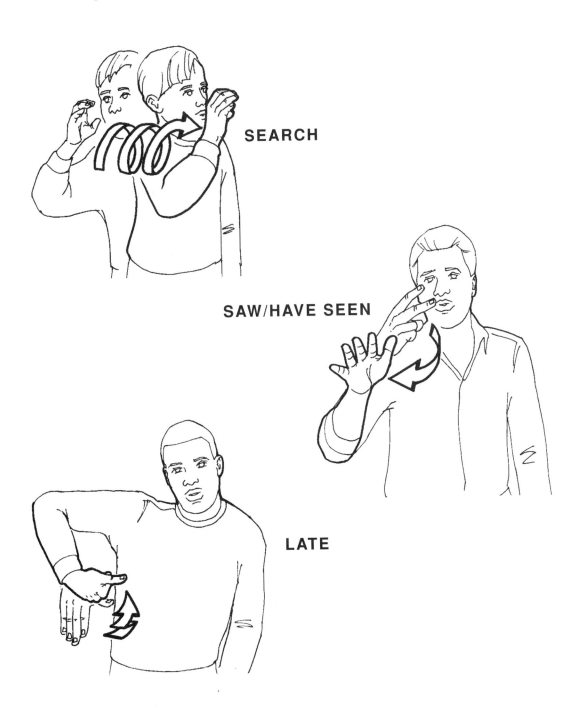

SEARCH

SAW/HAVE SEEN

LATE

- Suppose our mother and father want to go on a trip next year.
- Remember, tomorrow you and I will shop.
- Today in class we were excited to study sign language.
- I already watched that movie. I saw it late yesterday night.
- Look for the book where you put it yesterday.

Notice that the formal sign for "saw/have seen" is a contraction of the formal signs for "see" and "finished"; the signs have merged to create a more efficient, condensed movement.

We hope that you've had fun learning about Deaf culture and the Deaf experience while studying the basics of American Sign Language. In learning ASL, you acquire more than just the ability to use a new language: You discover an entirely new visual dimension of communication that will enrich *all* of your conversations. Whether signing in ASL or speaking in English, your ideas will take on an added depth of perception and feeling. Sign language teaches us to use our eyes, bodies, faces, hands, and emotions to express ourselves. A natural human language, it is the key that unlocks the power and beauty of visual communication.

EXERCISE

It is time to celebrate our first steps in learning the beautiful picture language of ASL. Have a party with your friends, Deaf and hearing, to share your experiences and newfound knowledge. Use the exercises throughout this book as party games to reinforce what you've studied, learn even more from your Deaf friends, and introduce hearing friends to the fun of natural gesture and sign language.

Putting It All Together

In a group, write words on cards and place them in a hat. Each person draws a card.

1. Start a conversation where each person in the room must add a sentence in sign language using the word or concept on the card they have. How long can you keep the conversation going?

2. Ask people to create "living" sentences in ASL word order by arranging themselves with the word-cards they are holding. Remember that ASL word order is different from the word order of an English sentence. Perform your sentences by having each person make the appropriate ASL sign in turn. You are communicating in three dimensions!

Additional Vocabulary

ARRIVE. Place the nondominant flat five-hand, fingers closed, across the body with the palm facing you. Take the dominant hand, in the same handshape, and move it from the chest to rest in the palm of the base hand. You have arrived.

BRIGHT. See "lamp" on page 98.

DARK. Place the fingertips of your flat five-hands, palms facing the body, in front of your temples. Bring the hands in a downward motion in front of the face, crossing the hands in front of the mouth to end with the fingertips pointing downward. You are shutting off the ability to see.

EARLY. Make a fist with the base hand, palm facing the floor and thumb facing the body. Place the dominant hand, palm facing down, over the base with fingers spread and pointing in front of you. Bend the middle finger at its middle joint and touch the fingertip to the back of the base hand; brush the fingertip across the back of the hand in an outward motion.

MINUTE. Begin at the starting point of the sign for "hour" (on page 144). From the wrist, rotate the extended pointer finger of the dominant hand slightly to the right, in a clockwise direction, to show a minute-hand ticking one minute.

SEASON. Hold the nondominant flat five-hand in front of you, palm facing out, to form a base, as in the sign for "minute." Make a fist with the dominant hand and lay it to touch the thumb and index finger side against the base palm; thumb points to the ceiling. From the wrist, rotate the fist in a clockwise direction. This shows the earth turning from one season to the next.

AUTUMN. Hold the nondominant flat five-hand, fingers closed, straight up like a tree. With the dominant five-hand, thumb in and palm facing down, brush the leaves off the tree.

SPRING. Place the nondominant hand in the "C" or "claw" handshape in front of the body. Bring the dominant hand underneath with thumb and fingertips pressed together. Push the thumb and fingertips through the open "C"-hand of the base and open them as they come through, the dominant palm faces your body. You are showing a flower blooming, or a plant growing. This is also the formal sign for "grow."

SUMMER. The index finger of the dominant hand moves across the eyebrow and crooks as it moves, as if you are wiping sweat from your brow.

WINTER. See "cold" on page 135.

The American Manual Alphabet

This classic rendition of the American Manual Alphabet depicts hand-shapes that denote letters. We have included the chart as a reference; it is necessary to understand that to spell individual letters on your hands—to fingerspell—can be tedious for lengthy conversations. For example, can you imagine speaking letters aloud to your hearing friends, "H-o-w   a-r-e   y-o-u   t-o-d-a-y   ?"

Deaf people prefer their full, rich American Sign Language (ASL) to communicate effectively. It is appropriate to spell out in handshapes proper nouns, places, and special terminology. This is similar to spoken English in that we might spell proper nouns for clarity. It is important to focus primarily on learning ASL because fingerspelling alone is merely a code for English. Understanding and executing letters spelled in the air requires advanced fine motor skills, which will be more readily acquired after acheiving fluency in ASL.

These engravings were made from photographs and printed in 1886; proving that Deaf Americans have been using ASL for over a hundred years. The letters of the English alphabet are listed on the cuf-flinks, corresponding to the letter of the manual alphabet each hand-shape depicts. The cufflinks could just as well have been pearl buttons on a woman's sleeve: Women, men, and their families were signing together at the beginning of the twentieth century—just as they are now as we begin the twenty-first century!

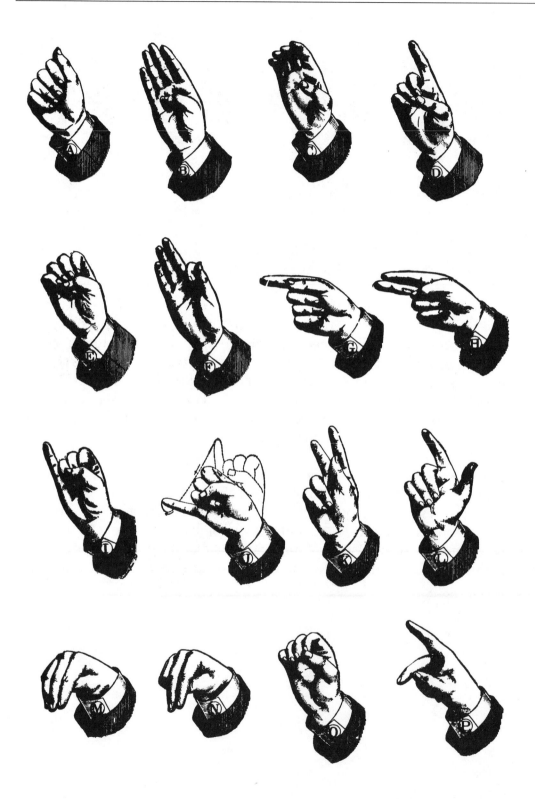

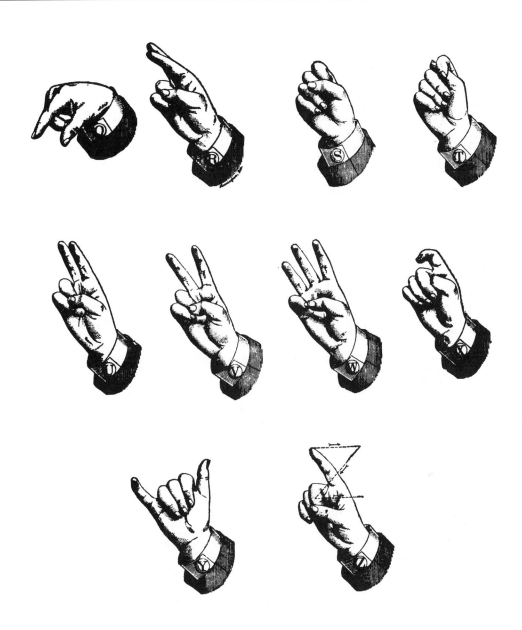

Suggested Reading

Baker, Charolotte and Robbin Battison, eds. *Sign Language in the Deaf Community: Essays in Honor of William Stokoe*. Silver Spring, MD: National Association of the Deaf, 1987.

Bragg, Bernard. *Lessons in Laughter* (as signed to Eugene Bergman). Washington, DC: Gallaudet University Press, 1989.

Cagle, Sharon, and Keith Cagle. *GA and SK Etiquette: Guidelines for Telecommunications in the Deaf Community*. Ohio: Bowling Green Press, Inc., 1991.

Cokely, Dennis, and Charlotte Baker. *American Sign Language*. Maryland: TJ Publishers, Inc., 1982.

Commission on Education of the Deaf. *Towards Equality: Education of the Deaf*. A Report to the President and the Congress of the United States, U.S. Government Printing Office, 1988.

Dolnick, E. 1993. "Deafness as Culture." *The Atlantic Monthly*, 272, 3.

Gallaudet Encyclopedia of Deaf and Deafness. New York: McGraw Hill, Inc., 1987.

Gannon, Jack. *Deaf Heritage: A Narrative History of Deaf America*. Silver Spring, MD: National Association of the Deaf, 1981.

———. *The Week the World Heard Gallaudet*. Washington, DC: Gallaudet University Press, 1989.

Groce, Norah Ellen. *Everyone Here Spoke Sign Language: Hereditary Deafness on Martha's Vineyard*. Massachusetts: Harvard University Press, 1985.

Humphrey, Janice, and Bob Alcorn. *So You Want to Be an Interpreter: An Introduction to Sign Language Interpreting*. Texas: H & H Publishers, 1985.

Jacobs, Leo. *A Deaf Adult Speaks Out.* Washington, DC: Gallaudet University Press, 1989.

Lane, Harlan. *When the Mind Hears.* New York: Random House, 1984.

Lane, Harlan, Robert Hoffmeister, and Ben Bahan. *A Journey into the Deaf World.* San Diego: Dawn Sign Press, 1996.

Meyers, Peter. *The ADA and You: A Guide for Deaf and Hard of Hearing People.* Washington, DC: The National Academy at Gallaudet University, 1992.

National Center for Law and Deafness. *Legal Rights: The Guide for Deaf and Hard of Hearing People.* Washington, DC: Gallaudet University Press, 1992.

Neisser, Arden. *The Other Side of Silence: Sign Language and the Deaf Community in America.* New York: Alfred A. Knopf, Inc., 1983.

President's Committee on Employment of People with Disabilities. *Employment Rights: Who Has Them and Who Enforces Them.* Washington, DC, 1994.

Sachs, Oliver. *Seeing Voices.* Berkley: University of California Press, 1989.

Smith, Sherri, Ella Mae Lentz, and Ken Mikos. Vista: *Signing Naturally.* San Diego: Dawn Sign Press, 1993.

Solomon, A. August 28, 1994. "Deaf Is Beautiful." *The New York Times Magazine.*

Wilcox, S., ed. *American Deaf Culture: An Anthology.* Silver Spring, MD: Linstok Press, 1989.

Woodward, J. and Markowicz, H. Language and the maintenance of ethnic boundaries in the deaf community. *How You Gonna Get to Heaven if You Can't Talk to Jesus: On Depathologizing Deafness.* Silver Spring, MD: TJ Publishers, Inc., 1982.

Resources

Alexander Graham Bell Association for
the Deaf
3417 Volta Place NW
Washington, DC 20007
202-337-5220 V/TTY
agbell2@aol.com

American Speech-Language-Hearing
Foundation
10801 Rockville Pike
Rockville, MD 20852
301-897-5700 V/TTY
foundation@asha.org

Catonsville Community College
Interpreter Preparation Program
800 South Rolling Rd.
Baltimore, MD 21228
410-455-6050 V

CJ Sign Language
14622 Ventura Blvd. #1010
Sherman Oaks, CA 91403
818-789-1348 Fax

Cleveland Hearing and Speech Center
Community Services for the Deaf
11206 Euclid Ave.
Cleveland, OH 44106
216-231-8787 V/TTY
216-231-7141 Fax

CUNY Consortium Interpreter Education
Project
250 Bedford Park Blvd. W
Bronx, NY 10468
718-960-6009 V
718-960-8744 TTY
718-960-8932 Fax

Deaf Culture Consulting
4527 South Dakota Ave. NE
Washington, DC 20017
202-635-0928 TTY
202-832-8078 Fax

Deaf Independent Living Association, Inc.
110 Baptist St.
PO Box 4038
Salisbury, MD 21803
410-742-5052 V/TTY
410-543-4874 Fax

Deaflife
PO Box 23380
Rochester, NY 14692-1788
716-442-6371 Fax

DeBee Communications
1709 South Braddock Ave.
Pittsburgh, PA 15218
619-931-9305 TTY
619-931-9222 Fax
http://www.debee.com

Equal Employment Opportunity Commission
1801 L Street NW
Washington, DC 20507
800-669-EEOC V
800-800-3302 TTY

Flying Hands
6400 Baltimore Baltimore National Pike, Ste. 103
Baltimore, MD 21228
410-788-6654 V/TTY
410-744-SIGN Fax

Gallaudet University
Sign Language and Professional Studies
Gallaudet University Kellogg Conference Center
800 Florida Ave. NE
Washington, DC 20002-3695
202-651-6057 V/TTY
202-651-6019 Fax

Harris Communications, Inc.
15159 Technology Dr.
Eden Prarie, MN 55344-2277
800-825-6758 V
800-825-9187 TTY
612-906-1099 Fax

The Hearing and Speech Agency
Centralized Interpreter Referral Service
2220 St. Paul St.
Baltimore, MD 21218
410-243-3800 V/TTY
410-243-1275 Fax

Hear-More Products
PO Box 3413
Farmingdale, NY 11735
800-881-4327 V/TTY
516-752-0689

Maryland School for the Deaf
101 Clarke Pl.
PO Box 250
Frederick, MD 21705-0250
301-620-8500 V
301-620-8555 TTY
frederick@msd.edu

MD Department of Budget and Management
Telecommunications Access of Maryland
301 West Preston St., Ste. 1008
Baltimore, MD 21201
800- 552-7274 V/TTY (in Maryland)
800-767-6960 V/TTY (from anywhere)
E Mail: moreinfo@mdrelay.org

NAD Broadcaster
814 Thayer Ave.
Silver Spring, MD 20910-4500
301-587-1788 V
301-587-1789 TTY

National Association of the Deaf
814 Thayer Ave.
Silver Spring, MD 20910-4500
301-587-1788 V
301-587-1789 TTY
nadhq@juno.com

National Center on Deafness
California State University, Northridge
18111 Nordhoff St.
Northridge, CA 91330-8267
818-885-2611 V/TTY
818-885-4899 Fax

National Information Center on Deafness
Gallaudet University
800 Florida Ave. NE
Washington, DC 20002-3695
202-651-5051 V
202-651-5052 TTY
mcoogan@gallua.gallaudet.edu

Nationwide Flashing Signal Systems
8120 Fenton St.
Silver Spring, MD 20910
301-589-5153 V
301-589-6670 TTY

Nexion, Inc.
3191 South Valley St., Ste. 205
Salt Lake City, UT 84109
810-466-1258 V
810-466-0453 TTY
810-466-1259 Fax
nxi@nxicom.com

NTID/RIT Department for ASL and Interpreting
Education
52 Lomb Memorial Dr.
Rochester, NY 14623-5604
716-475-6431 V/TTY
716-475-6500 Fax

Phone-TTY, Inc.
202 Lexington Ave.
Hackensack, NJ 07601-4043
201-489-7889 V
201-489-7890 TTY
201-489-7891 Fax

Potomac Technology
One Church St., Ste. 101
Rockville, MD 20850
800-433-2838 V/TTY
301-762-4005 V/TTY
301-762-0851 V/TTY
301-762-1892 Fax

The Registry of Interpreters for the Deaf, Inc.
8630 Fenton ST STE 324
Silver Spring, MD 20910-3919
301-608-0050 V
301-608-0562 TTY
301-608-0508 Fax

Robertson Communications, Inc.
One Chancery Ct.
Reisterstown, MD 21136
410-526-1312 Fax
Drobert364@aol.com

Self Help for Hard of Hearing People Inc.
7910 Woodmont Ave., Ste. 1200
Bethesda, MD 20814
301-657-2248 V
301-657-2249 TTY
national@shhh.org

Sign Enhancers, Inc.
1535 State St.
Salem, OR 97301-4255
800-767-4461 V/TTY
503-370-6457 Fax
sigen@aol.com

Sign Media, Inc.
4020 Blackburn Ln.
Burtonsville, MD 20866
301-421-0268 V/TTY

Silent News, Inc.
1425 Jefferson Rd.
Rochester, NY 14623-3139

Telecommunications Access of Maryland
State of Maryland Budget and Management
301 West Preston St., Ste. 1008
Baltimore, MD 21201
410-767-5891 V/TTY
800-552-7724 V/TTY
410-767-4276 Fax

TJ Publishers
817 Silver Spring Ave., Ste. 206
Silver Spring, MD 20910-4617
800-999-1168 V/TTY
301-585-5930 Fax

TRIPOD
2901 N. Keystone St.
Burbank, CA 91504
818-972-2080 V/TTY
818-972-2090 Fax

US Department of Justice
Civil Rights Division
Office on the Americans with Disabilities Act
PO Box 66118
Washington, DC 20035-6118
202-514-0301 V
202-514-0383 TTY

Western Maryland College
Office of Graduate Studies
2 College Hill
Westminster, MD 21157-4390
410-876-2055 V
410-857-2773 Fax

Index of Signs

Our eyes are our ears; our hands are our voices.
—Quote from the Deaf community

Note: Page numbers designated with a "d" indicate signs used in dialogues. Page numbers designated with an "f" indicate figures.